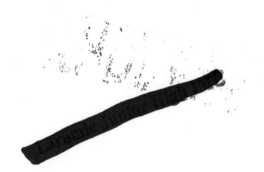

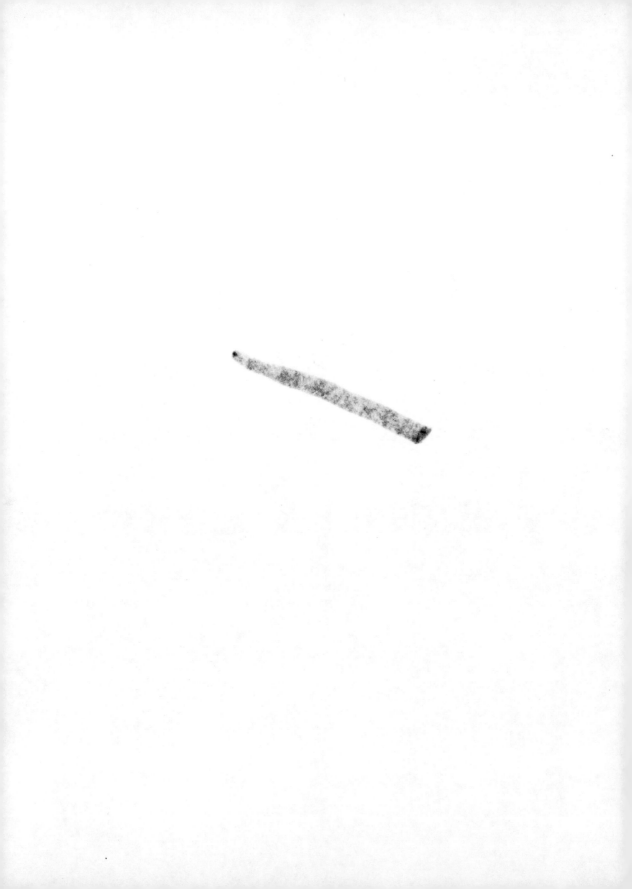

LEGENDS OF HEALTH & FITNESS

# Female Stars of Nutrition and Weight Control

featuring profiles of
Suzanne Somers, Oprah Winfrey,
Nadia Comaneci, and Marilu Henner

Susan Zannos

Mitchell Lane Publishers, Inc.
PO Box 619
Bear, DE 19701

# LEGENDS OF HEALTH & FITNESS

## Role Models for Young Adults
## Who Want to Lead a Healthy and Fit Lifestyle

MITCHELL LANE PUBLISHERS, INC.

# WHY DO WE CARE ABOUT HEALTH & FITNESS?

Do you remember the old adage that goes, "If you don't have your health, you have nothing at all?" When we are young, we think we are immortal. We think we are invincible. We will never get sick, grow old, or die. But, as we get older, we become more aware of our mortality. We realize that we can't enjoy life if we are not healthy. We can't go to work every day and earn a living. We get tired on short walks or winded walking up stairs. We are only on this earth for a short while, and to live life to its fullest, we must make sure we stay healthy and fit.

Healthy habits begin early in life. We need exercise and good nutrition every day. Millions of people have adopted daily workout routines and nutritious, healthy eating habits. Among these millions are some very famous people, who despite their very active lives, make time each day to ensure their health and fitness. They come from many different careers and backgrounds. In this series, we have put together profiles of forty fitness role models whose dedication to health and fitness complement their life and career. Hopefully, you will make the same commitment to health and fitness that these people have made and as a result, will enjoy a long, happy, and healthy life.

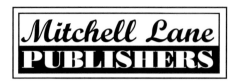

*Mitchell Lane*
**PUBLISHERS**

First Printing

Library of Congress Cataloging-in-Publication Data
Zannos, Susan.
     Female Stars of Nutrition and Weight Control : featuring profiles of Suzanne Somers, Oprah Winfrey, Nadia Comaneci and Marilu Henner / Susan Zannos.
        p. cm.—(Legends of health & fitness)
     Includes bibliographical references and index.
     ISBN 1-58415-015-7
     1. Weight loss—Juvenile literature. 2. Henner, Marilu—Juvenile literature. 3. Winfrey, Oprah—Juvenile literature. 4. Comaneci, Nadia, 1961—Juvenile literature. 5. Somers, Suzanne, 1946—Juvenile literature. 6. Nutritionists—Biography—Juvenile literature. 7. Television personalities—Biography—-Juvenile literature. [1. Television personalities 2. Actors and actresses. 3. Physical fitness.] I. Title. II. Series
RM222.2 .Z36 2000
613.2'092'273—dc21
[B]
                                            00-031626

**About the Author:** Susan Zannos has taught at all levels, from preschool to college, in Mexico, Greece, Italy, Russia, and Lithuania, as well as in the United States. She has published a mystery *Trust the Liar* (Walker and Co.) and *Human Types: Essence and the Enneagram* was published by Samuel Weiser in 1997. She has written several books for children, including *Paula Abdul* and *Cesar Chavez* (Mitchell Lane).
**Photo Credits:** pp. 6, 14 Superstock; p. 18 Shooting Star; p. 25 The Kobal Collection; p. 28 Shooting Star; p. 32 The Kobal Collection; p. 34 Shooting Star; p. 38 Globe Photos; p. 49 Archive Photos; p. 50 Shooting Star; p. 52 AP Photo; p. 54 Globe Photos; p. 58 Globe Photos; pp. 64, 65 Allsport; pp. 71, 73 Globe Photos; p. 76 Archive Photos; p. 82 AP Photos; pp. 87, 89, 90 Shooting Star
**Acknowledgments:** The following stories have been thoroughly researched. To the best of our knowledge, they represent true stories. While every possible effort has been made to ensure accuracy, the publisher will not assume liability for damages caused by inaccuracies in the data, and makes no warranty on the accuracy of the information contained herein. None of the stories have been authorized or endorsed by the people we have profiled. The story on Marilu Henner has been reviewed and approved for print by her representatives.

# Table of Contents

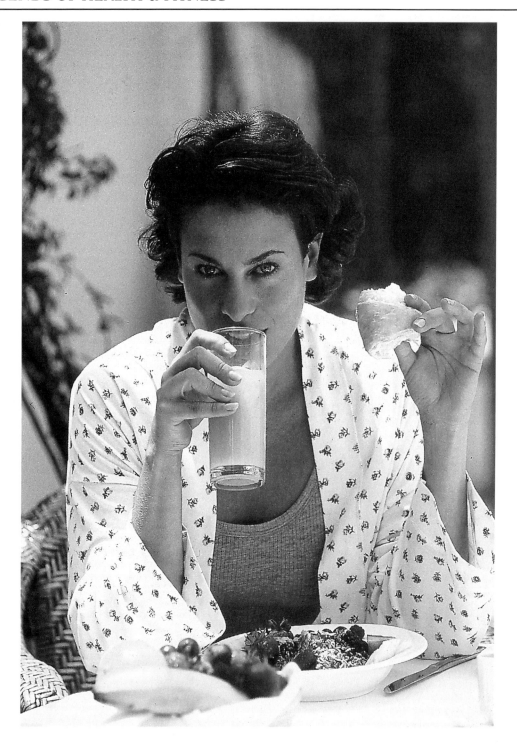

*For good health, combine a healthy diet with a regular exercise routine.*

# CHAPTER ONE
# Healthy Living

**A**ccording to the U.S. Surgeon General, obesity is one of our country's most serious health problems. More than 20 percent of children and 50 percent of all Americans are overweight. By improving nutritional habits and increasing physical activity, Americans can reduce the occurrence of several life-threatening illnesses, such as heart disease and some types of cancer.

Obesity—too much fat stored in the body—is a complex problem, and one with which Americans seem to be obsessed. Thousands of books have been published that claim to present the perfect weight-loss diet. Almost every magazine available on newsstands today advertises a weight-loss plan on its cover. Many of the same magazine covers feature photos of models and movie stars who are so thin that their bones are nearly visible through their skin. The ideal image of beauty is a fat-free body—while at the same time, most real bodies are getting fatter and fatter.

Losing excess weight is not easy. One of the biggest obstacles is dieting. Dieting can actually cause weight gain. The metabolism, which is the regulating device that determines how rapidly the body expends energy, gradually slows down as a person consumes less food. For our ancestors thousands of years ago, this metabolic phenomenon was a very important key to survival. It was so important in helping people live through periods of famine and through harsh winters when food was scarce, that the ones who ultimately survived were those who had the genetic programming to store fat efficiently—in other words, those whose metabolisms would slow down dramatically as they ate less. These ancestors, of course, passed down their genes to their children and grandchildren, and eventually to us.

Not only does the metabolism slow down when one is dieting, but when the dieter stops restricting food intake the body begins rapidly storing fat again—and very frequently it ends up storing more fat than it started with. The result is a desperate cycle of weight loss and gain, in which an overweight person may gain even more as he or she tries harder to lose it.

For this reason, many of the so-called miracle diets we read about today may actually cause fast weight loss at first—but in the long run they are doomed to fail. Such diets usually consist of odd and very restrictive food combinations that would ruin the health of anyone who continued the diet longer than a few weeks. Or the diet may rely on supplements and drugs. After the dieter resumes eating normal balanced meals, however, his or her body will most likely react by gaining weight rapidly.

Does this mean that it is impossible to diet to lose weight? Not at all. What it does mean is that losing weight and keeping the weight off are not easy. It means that when a diet claims to be easy—to guarantee a loss of 10 to 20 pounds in 10 days, for example—it is probably a setup for eventual weight gain, not loss.

Unfortunately, there really is no quick and easy solution for weight loss. The only long-term solution to weight control is to change permanently the factors in one's life that have helped to add the weight in the first place. To take weight off and then go back to the same behaviors that caused weight gain will not help. Albert Einstein once described insanity as "Endlessly repeating the same process, hoping for a different result." Are most dieters insane? Surely not, but the hope of finding a quick fix for weight gain certainly is!

What one eats is only one of the factors a person needs to change when attempting to lose weight. One of the most important ways of staying fit and controlling weight gain is to engage in regular exercise. The solution is not easy or fast, but it makes sense: if the body takes in more food than it can convert into energy, then the excess will be stored as fat. So while you can simply control your food intake and lose weight, you are even more likely to do so when you combine a healthy diet with an exercise routine.

One of the reasons Americans have become increasingly overweight in this century is that while high-calorie, high-fat convenience foods have become more popular, we have also become more sedentary. Most of us will take a car instead of walking to our destination, and at work we most likely sit at a desk or computer rather than perform physical labor. Exactly how to change eating habits to meet nutritional needs while burning excess body fat varies from person to person. No single system works for everyone, regardless of what all the diet books and videotapes say. Nonetheless, some general guidelines are useful when undertaking any weight-loss plan.

In a balanced diet, three main categories of foods are necessary in varying amounts: proteins, carbohydrates, and fats. Any diet plan that requires completely eliminating one of these categories is doomed to eventual failure, so it makes a lot more sense to embark on a reasonable eating plan right from the start. However, some foods in each category can be eliminated, or at least restricted, with little or no loss of nutritional benefits. That's because some foods have little nutritional value to begin with.

The energy units available from food are called calories, and many diets simply limit the number of calories that one consumes each day. But it's also important to regulate the kind of calories one is consuming. Virtually all nutritionists agree that calories from highly processed carbohydrates, such as sugar and white flour, are more likely to be stored as fat than used for energy, so they are usually the first to be eliminated from a sensible diet plan. Other kinds of carbohydrates, such as those available in fruits, vegetables and whole grains, are healthier for the body because they are digested more slowly and the energy is used over a longer period of time. If you eat a food that is high in processed carbohydrates, such as a doughnut, you may feel an immediate burst of energy—but an hour later the energy will have been spent, and you will probably feel tired or hungry again. On the other hand, if you eat a piece of whole wheat toast instead of a doughnut, you will maintain a more steady energy level over a longer period.

Protein is available from meat, fish, eggs, dairy products, and some kinds of vegetables, such as soybeans. Nutritionists seem to agree that proteins from fish and the white meat of chicken and turkey are the most desirable types. They also agree that it is better to consume as little animal fat as possible with the protein; as a result, many recommend avoiding fatty meats and fried foods.

Fats and oils from vegetable sources, including olive oil, canola oil, and peanut oil, are preferred to animal fats such as butter because they do not contain cholesterol. Beyond that, however, there are widely varying opinions about the recommended levels of fats in a healthful diet. Some nutritionists recommend severely restricting fat intake; others strongly disagree and believe that consuming too many carbohydrates is responsible for most weight gain. It seems that fats that are consumed are used by the body before it resorts to stored fats. Thus, consuming a lot of fat seems to be counterproductive for someone on a weight-loss diet. But the body's way of generating energy is much more complicated, so the controversy over the proper fat levels in a healthy diet continues.

In the United States, all food packagers are now legally required to include nutritional information on the labels of all their products. A quick scan of one of these labels can tell you the number of calories, the percentages of fat, carbohydrate, and protein, and the percentage of nutritional elements such as vitamins and minerals in each serving of the product. Unfortunately, although such information is easily available, what we should do with the information is still unclear at times. Experts of varying degrees have written scores of books and articles about weight control, and each "plan" is based on a different theory about what constitutes a healthful diet. So much seemingly contradictory information is available that it is easy for a person who is trying to lose weight to become discouraged before he or she even begins a weight-loss program. One diet plan might insist that the key to successful weight loss is to eliminate all fat from the diet; another will declare that some fat is necessary. One plan will completely eliminate carbohydrates, while another might severely restrict protein consumption. Some nutritional experts provide extremely detailed outlines of what constitutes a "balanced" meal, and warn that any deviation will hinder one's success. Others insist that the key to losing weight is to eat different kinds of foods separately—to eat only fruit at one meal, only carbohydrates at another meal, and only proteins at a third meal, for example.

Not only is what to eat in question, but also when to eat it. Some experts say to eat only three daily meals, while others suggest that eating five or six small meals each day is more beneficial. Some tell us that we should eat only when we feel hungry; others say we should eat according to a schedule, whether we feel hungry or not. Still others suggest that it is even better to eat when not hungry. One school of thought recommends eating nothing after 6:00 P.M. Another recommends having a snack before going to bed so that the body will have some fuel through the long fasting period before breakfast.

How is it possible that so much disagreement exists among nutritional, medical, and physical fitness authorities? One probable reason is that every individual is different. Some fortunate people seem to be able to eat anything they want in whatever quantities they want without ever putting on weight. These people are blessed with good metabolisms that "burn off" calories more efficiently than others. Then again, some people have efficient metabolisms, but very bad eating habits. Maybe they gain weight, but they may also find it easy to take off and keep off once they make a few minor adjustments in their diet, such as substituting low-fat items for their favorite foods or skipping sugary desserts.

Some researchers have suggested that even those who have great difficulty losing weight may have those difficulties for varying reasons, and nutritionists have devised systems that are tailored to different types. One such system suggests that in each person, a different endocrine gland may be most active, and that it is the dominant gland that determines the type of diet required for that person to lose weight. A person with active adrenal glands, for example, may need more protein than other types, while one with a more active pancreas does better when whole grains are the foundation of the diet. Another recently advertised program maintains that one's diet should be based on blood type. The theory is that the bodies of people of different ethnic—and therefore genetic—backgrounds are predisposed to handle certain kinds of food more efficiently, and therefore their diets need to be tailored to the foods most suitable for them.

But whatever the latest nutritional theory may be, most diets can be classified into these categories:

- Fat-burning diets that rely on a few specific foods
- Calorie-restrictive diets that eliminate fats and other high-calorie foods
- "Balanced" diets that prescribe exactly how much of each food group to consume
- Combining diets that require eating different types of food at different meals

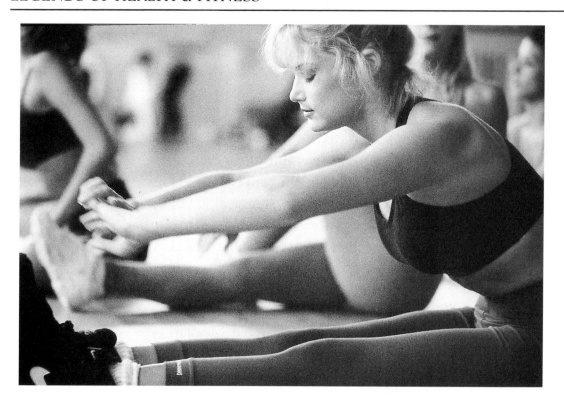

*A regular fitness program will help you achieve your weight-loss goal.*

While many diets may include elements of several categories, most eating plans rely primarily on one of them alone.

The first of these, the so-called fat-burning diets, should be viewed with great caution. Examples of this kind of diet would be the Mayo Diet (which has no connection with the famous Mayo Clinic). This diet is also referred to as the "grapefruit and egg diet" because it is based mainly on consuming protein and grapefruit. Very similar to the Mayo Diet are the "meat and oranges diet" and the diet proposed in books by Dr. Robert Atkins. These are diets that require eating mostly proteins, with some acidic (citrus) fruits and occasional green vegetables.

These diets work by changing the body's chemistry to a state called ketosis, in which fat, and unfortunately also lean muscle, is burned very rapidly. Ketosis can be measured by testing the urine for ketones with special strips available in pharmacies. In this way, Atkins believes, it is possible to induce some ketosis without allowing it to get out of control (it is a potentially dangerous condition). In general, it is not wise to interfere with the body's natural chemical balance. While ketogenic diets certainly can cause quite rapid weight loss, they may cause weight gain in the long run when the body attempts to compensate. At the other extreme are diets that prescribe eating nothing but carbohydrates, and frequently only one or two kinds, such as brown rice. Macrobiotic diets would be included in this category. They eliminate all proteins and fats.

The second category, the calorie-restrictive diets, approach weight loss by focusing on calorie counting. The most extreme of these programs include complete or partial fasts and rely on vitamin and mineral supplements to replace the nutrients lost during fasting. The obvious drawback to such diets is that dieters who follow the program do not learn to change their eating habits permanently. Once they end a fasting period and begin eating regularly again, they nearly always gain back the weight they lost—and sometimes they gain even more. Other calorie- restricting diets provide specific lists of foods and their caloric values and recommend eating nothing but what is on the list. Foods such as lettuce and celery, which are extremely low in calories, are highly recommended, but if the dieter chooses to consume, say, all of his or her 800 daily calories by eating one piece of chocolate cake, that's fine, too. The primary obstacle to this type of diet is the body's own way of defending itself against fasting: the

fewer calories consumed, the fewer the body will release as energy. The metabolism slows down, and weight
gain often results.

The third type of program, the so-called balanced
diets, are the most moderate of weight-loss programs.
But even in this category, opinions differ strongly about
exactly what constitutes a "balance." Most of the group
weight-loss programs, such as Weight Watchers, Jenny
Craig, and Diet Center, follow carefully balanced diets.
Weight Watchers, for example, adheres to the U.S.
Department of Agriculture (USDA) food pyramid as the
basis for its diets. Other proponents of balanced diet
programs—such as Barry Sears, who developed the
"Zone Diet"— disagree with USDA recommendations
and propose their own balance. For example, while the
USDA advises consuming roughly four times as many
carbohydrates as proteins daily, Sears recommends consuming approximately equal amounts, making sure that
the carbohydrates are in fruits and vegetables.

The fourth category of food programs, combination diets, are similar to the balanced diets with one
main difference: while most combination diets recommend consuming a variety of foods, they advise that
you consume them separately. The unproven theory
behind this is that the digestive system works more efficiently when it processes one type of food at a time.
Therefore, fruits, proteins, and carbohydrates are consumed separately, several hours apart. Well-known
combination diets, such as the "Hollywood Diet," which
focuses on tropical fruits such as mangoes and papa-
yas, have been quite popular and are seemingly effec-
tive. The problem with combination diets is that they
are difficult to sustain. Most people have trouble stick-
ing to such a diet when their lives include grabbing quick

meals during business days, dining out, attending parties and social occasions, and having dinner with the rest of the family who do not follow the diet.

The vast array of weight-loss programs and the overwhelming amount of nutritional information available today teach us one important lesson: those who want to achieve fitness and lose weight must do their homework. You may have to experiment with several types of diets before you find the one that works best for you. In the end, though, another fact becomes clear: a healthy diet consisting of a variety of foods, combined with a regular fitness program, can help just about anyone achieve his or her goal.

In this book, we'll examine the ways in which four famous women—actress Suzanne Somers, entertainer Oprah Winfrey, former Olympic gymnast Nadia Comaneci, and actress Marilu Henner—have managed to achieve their nutritional goals. After years of struggle, each of them has found the solution to maintaining her weight and leading a healthy life.

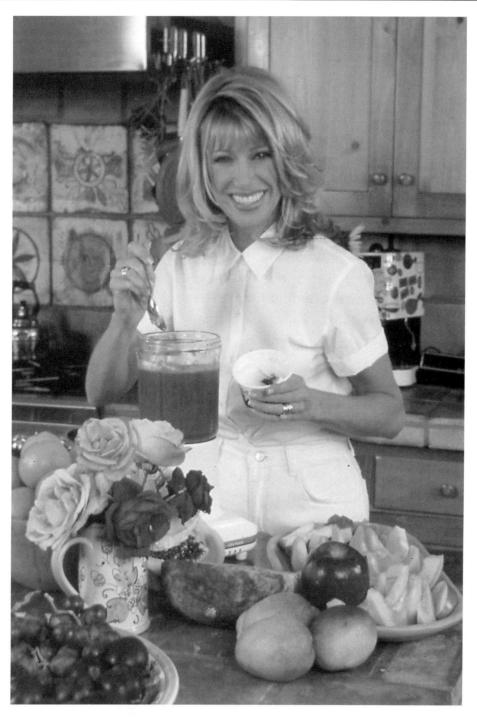

*Suzanne Somers has always enjoyed cooking.*

# CHAPTER TWO
## Suzanne Somers

When Suzanne Somers first moved to Los Angeles at the beginning of her show business career, she landed a role in the popular television series *Starsky and Hutch*—or so she thought. She had hoped that the opportunity would be the big break she needed to launch a career in television. But even before filming started, she received a call from the show's producer telling her that she didn't have the job after all. They had decided, he told her, that she was "a little too chunky" for the part.

Suzanne was devastated. Determined to land another role on a TV program, she began experimenting with all kinds of diets. "Guess what?" she now says. "They all worked. That's right. Every time I went on a diet, I lost weight. But within a short time of going back to eating like a normal person, I would gain back all the weight and often a little extra." This cycle of losing and gaining weight continued for years. Suzanne had always loved to cook. One of her chief delights was preparing delicious meals for her husband and their children—but at the same time, controlling her weight was absolutely necessary for her career. As she grew older and her metabolism slowed, the roller coaster of loss and gain changed somewhat. Now the weight came off more slowly and was more difficult to lose, while it became discouragingly easy for her to gain weight.

In other areas of her life, Suzanne Somers had learned the hard way that she could not escape her problems or pretend that they didn't exist. Several members of her family, including her father, suffered from the disease of alcoholism, and while Suzanne was growing up she knew what it was like to live a lie, to pretend to outsiders that everything was fine, when in reality her life was filled with insecurity, fear, and violence.

Suzanne was born on October 16, 1946, the third child of Frank and Marion Mahoney. A former baseball player, Frank worked in a brewery. He was a popular man, and he always seemed to be the life the party in any gathering. "I grew up thinking that all 'dads' got drunk," Suzanne remembers. "Of course, I couldn't understand alcoholism at this age. All I knew was [that my father] smelled bad, talked real loud, and played rough if he drank too much." As Frank Mahoney's disease worsened, he became more difficult to live with, and the Mahoney household was filled with constant fighting. And because Marion Mahoney was a devout Catholic, she could not imagine leaving or divorcing her husband, no matter how bad his behavior became.

At the time, few people were aware that alcoholism was a disease. Most people, including many medical experts, believed it was a problem of will power, and that anyone who truly wished to stop drinking could do so simply by putting his or her mind to it. We now know that it is a much more complicated problem than that—alcoholism is more of an addiction than a failure of will. We are also more aware today that alcoholism affects not only the person who has the disease but also that person's family and friends. Suzanne remembers that she and her brother and sister would sometimes hide in a closet when they heard their father coming home. They hoped that he would be too drunk to think of looking for them there. The children's fear of his outbursts was so strong that the three of them vowed that they would never drink alcohol when they grew up.

In 1957, when Suzanne was 11 years old, her father broke his heel while coaching a boys' baseball team, and he had to stay home from work for several months. It was a wonderful time for the family because Frank Mahoney wasn't able to go out drinking. During this period, Marion Mahoney worked while Frank kept up with the housekeeping. For a while, Suzanne felt like she was living in a normal family. Then her mother became pregnant with the Mahoneys' youngest child, Michael.

Eventually, of course, Frank's foot healed, and he returned to work at the brewery, where the temptation of being around alcohol overpowered him. The nights of drunken violence began once more, and Suzanne retreated to her closet. Her older brother and sister, meanwhile, grew more and more anxious to get out of the house and away from the suffering. In June 1959, Suzanne's sister Maureen married her high school sweetheart. A year later, her brother Danny joined the Navy. That left Suzanne and her two-year-old brother Michael alone with their parents in the little white house that was well-kept on the outside but concealed horrors inside.

Without the support of her older siblings, Suzanne felt isolated, and she retreated not only into her closet but also into her own fantasies. She dreamed of a life away from her parents' home, where she would be successful, wealthy, and popular. After Suzanne finished eighth grade her mother went back to work so that she could afford to enroll her daughter in an exclusive Catholic girls' school. No one at the school knew that Suzanne Mahoney's father was the "town drunk," and Suzanne tried to keep it that way. But the school had high academic standards, and the chaos at home prevented Suzanne from studying and getting enough sleep. Under pressure to keep up her grades, she started cheating at her schoolwork.

Most of Suzanne's classmates came from wealthy families, but since the girls all wore uniforms, they didn't know that the Mahoney family was not well off. Marion helped her daughter buy a few nice outfits to wear on special occasions, but when Frank Mahoney saw Suzanne wearing one of them one day he became enraged. He yanked the rest of the outfits from Suzanne's closet and tore them to pieces. And when Suzanne began dating, she and her mother devised a system in which her dates would not have to meet her drunken father. Suzanne would watch from the window and signal her mother when the boy arrived. Her mother would then distract her father long enough to give Suzanne time to slip out of the house.

One of the fantasies Suzanne indulged in was writing love letters to a boy for whom she had developed a crush. She never intended to send the notes, but when a nun found the letters in Suzanne's locker at school, she expelled the girl. Only a few weeks from finishing her sophomore year, Suzanne enrolled in the local public high school, where she was relieved to find that the schoolwork was much less demanding. There, she also tried out for the school play, a production of the Broadway musical *Guys and Dolls,* and she earned one of the leading roles.

At the time, Suzanne was dating Bruce Somers, a student at the University of San Francisco. When she graduated from high school in June 1964 with a $500 music scholarship, she was accepted at Lone Mountain College, an all-female Catholic college just across the street from the university. Suzanne's high school grades weren't the best, but she had invented a fascinating story about herself to include on the college application form, and the school had accepted her in part based on the background she'd made up. To help pay her tuition, she found a job selling dresses. Suzanne reveled in the elegant atmosphere of Lone Mountain. Most of all, she loved being away from home, even though she felt pangs of guilt over leaving her mother and younger brother alone with her father.

Although Suzanne dated others, she felt most comfortable with Bruce, the one friend who knew about her family situation. She enjoyed going out with Bruce, even though he sometimes became overly amorous after fraternity parties, where he would usually drink heavily. One night, Bruce took Suzanne back to her dorm after the doors had been locked. Unable to get back into the building, Suzanne took a hotel room with Bruce for the night. Shortly afterwards, Suzanne realized that she was pregnant.

Suzanne's Catholic upbringing led her to believe that the only solution was to marry Bruce. She knew that she did not love him, but on April 14, 1965, Suzanne and Bruce were married. "I couldn't believe it," she remembers. "Monday, just another college girl; Thursday, a pregnant married woman." Their son, named Bruce for his father, was born on November 8, 1965. Suzanne adored her son, but she knew that she was not ready to have more children. So despite her desire to follow the teachings of the Catholic Church, she began taking birth control pills.

Suzanne felt trapped and miserable in her marriage. Bruce worked all day and studied at night. After he graduated from college, he entered law school. To get out of their small apartment and earn extra income, Suzanne took a job as a nurse's aide at a nearby hospital. Every weekday she worked from 2 to 5 P.M., came home to feed the baby and prepare dinner, and then returned to the hospital until 10 P.M. But the routine and the stress gnawed at her: at just 18 years old, Suzanne began to feel as though her life was over.

One day she impulsively began an affair with one of her former college teachers. She didn't have the courage to ask Bruce for a divorce—she knew what her family would say—so she began seeing the man after work at night. She lied to Bruce, telling him that things were so busy at the hospital that she had to work until after midnight. But one night Bruce went to the hospital to see her and discovered that she wasn't there. The former teacher arrived at the Somers's apartment and tried to force Suzanne to leave her husband and marry him. Angry and hurt, Bruce took the baby and left his wife.

Not knowing where her child was instilled panic in Suzanne, but because of her affair she received no support from her family—not even from her mother. Although she repeatedly called her parents to find out whether they knew where Bruce had taken the baby, they refused to talk to her. Finally, Bruce returned (he had been staying at Suzanne's brother's house). Suzanne and Bruce decided that they would try to save their marriage.

The couple moved with their son to another town, where they rented a small house. Bruce was still working and going to school, and Suzanne got a job as a cocktail waitress. After several months, however, they both realized that the marriage wasn't working, and they agreed to divorce. Suzanne received custody of young Bruce. Now she was on her own with a child to support.

Nothing in Suzanne's background had prepared her for the responsibility of being a single mother. All she had known while growing up was the necessity of lying and denying reality in an effort to cope with her father's alcoholism. Though she was no longer in that situation, the denials persisted, even among the other members of her family. They never asked Suzanne how she was doing, or even where she was living, because they had difficulty accepting that she was divorced and on her own.

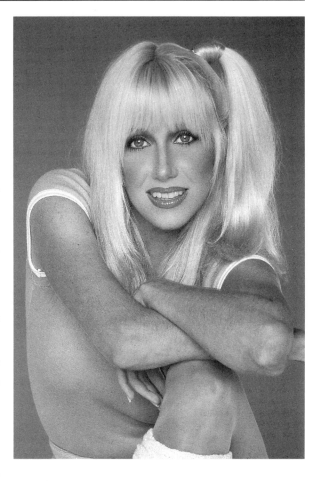

*Suzanne worked as a model in San Francisco to support her young son.*

Meanwhile, her sister Maureen and her brother Danny had succumbed to alcoholism as well. Suzanne watched in horror as the siblings with whom she had hidden in the closet—and with whom she had vowed never to drink—became more and more like their father. At family dinners, both Maureen and Danny would drink alcohol while their children and other family members ate. Before long, the two siblings would become loud and nasty, cursing and saying cruel things to their family members, just as their father had done with them while they were growing up. The next day, Maureen and Danny might feel guilty and remorseful— or worse, they might not even remember what they had said and done. Michael, Suzanne's younger brother, was especially under siege: he was the only one still living at home, and the only one who still had to withstand his father's drunken attacks, in addition to the vicious behavior of Maureen and Danny.

What Suzanne did not understand, because she was not drinking, was that she too was suffering from the family disease. For her, however, the uncontrollable drinking of other family members was not causing the crises and chaos in her life. Instead, it was her habit of denying reality, a defense mechanism that she had developed to cope with her family's alcoholism. It kept her from being responsible with her money, and it kept her from developing a healthy sense of self-respect.

Through a modeling agency, Suzanne had gotten a few jobs, including some work as an extra in movies and some bit parts in television commercials. But she didn't earn enough to cover her living expenses, and when she did get paid for a job, she could never resist going on a shopping spree and buying expensive clothing instead of paying her bills. When stores or collection agencies pressured her to pay up, she would write checks, blindly hoping that somehow she would get enough money in her bank account to cover them. She lived in a constant state of panic and crisis, never realizing that this was exactly the way she had lived at home with her father. It seemed that this was the only way she knew how to live.

But this way of life could not continue forever. In the summer of 1970, Suzanne Somers was arrested and jailed, charged with fraud for writing bad checks.

She called a lawyer she knew, who was able to convince the judge at her hearing that she was not a criminal, but simply young and inexperienced in handling money matters. The lawyer won her release. Suzanne borrowed money from friends to cover the bad checks and pay the lawyer.

Two years earlier, Suzanne had begun dating Alan Hamel, a TV show host whom she had met at a studio in San Francisco while on a modeling job. The two were immediately attracted to one another. Suzanne lied to Alan about her situation, however: she told him that her father had been a wealthy doctor who had left her a sizeable inheritance upon his death. She feared that if she told this powerful and attractive man the truth, he would reject her. That one lie led to many others, however, and she ended up constantly scrambling to hide her desperate financial situation from Alan.

Eventually, Suzanne discovered that Alan was married. Yet she continued to see him. At the time, she thought so little of herself that she believed he would refuse to see her if she objected to his lies about being married. As a result, she tried not to demand anything from him, and she pretended that she felt independent and enjoyed her freedom. In reality, she lived in terror that he would never call her again.

Suzanne began living a double life. When she traveled to Toronto, Los Angeles, or New York City to work with Alan, or when the two of them took exotic vacations, she missed her son terribly and felt guilty about leaving him with a neighbor or her mother. When she stayed at home with Bruce, however, she missed Alan and spent much of her time waiting for him to call. Finally, in December 1971, the situation came to a head.

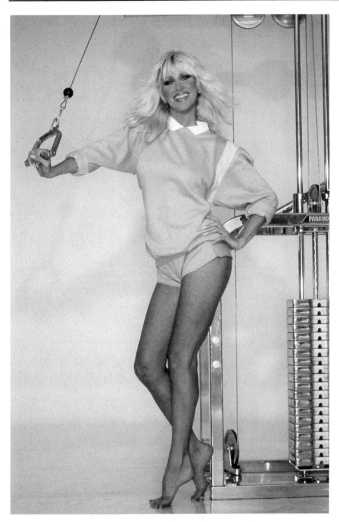

*A regular routine of exercise complements Suzanne's food combining plan.*

Alan was looking through Suzanne's Christmas cards one evening while she was fixing dinner for them. He discovered one that was signed "Mom and Dad," and confronted Suzanne about her story that her father was dead. Panicking, Suzanne began to make up yet another lie, explaining that her mother had refused to accept her father's death and still insisted on signing both of their names. Alan didn't believe her. Finally, Suzanne began to cry, and the whole truth about her parents spilled out of her. Alan had known for some time that something wasn't quite right with Suzanne, and both of them felt relieved to have the truth out in the open. But Suzanne still hadn't told Alan about her financial situation. He would find out about her second lie after an accident that very nearly became a tragedy.

Young Bruce was outside playing on a scooter his father had given him for Christmas when he was run over by a car. Suzanne rushed her son to the hospital, where he spent hours in surgery. At first, his doctors could not say for sure whether he would survive, but he eventually recovered. The medical bills, however, completely ruined Suzanne's chances of financial stability. She had nowhere to turn for the money she needed: Bruce Somers had never paid any child support, and he had told her that he couldn't even see the boy because he was trying to save his second marriage.

Even after little Bruce was home from the hospital, he had terrible nightmares. The bill collectors were harassing Suzanne every day. Meanwhile, she couldn't find work, and she spent most nights awake and comforting her screaming son. Finally, Suzanne turned to the local community center, which offered mental health counseling. A therapist agreed to see both Suzanne and her son weekly for an hour-long session each—and for only one dollar per session. Today, she is extremely grateful for the help. "It changed our lives," she says.

Gradually, the therapist caused Suzanne to question the way she was living. "You have to deal with this compulsive buying problem," the therapist told her. "It's unrealistic! On one hand, you tell me you don't have enough money for food, and then you tell me you spent $1,500 on clothes." Suzanne insisted that she needed the clothes for her work, and the therapist would ask if she had a plan for getting out of debt. Later Suzanne said, "She was trying to give me a framework on which to live. I needed a grasp on reality. I needed to recognize my worth as a human being."

The therapist also questioned Suzanne's relationship with Alan Hamel, and asked her why she asked so little of him. Suzanne began examining that aspect of her life, too. Gradually she developed more self-confidence and began to believe that she could achieve her dream of becoming an actress. After a year, the therapist declared that Bruce Jr. had recovered, but that Suzanne needed to continue her sessions. Suzanne would also begin paying more for each session—a way

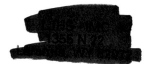

of proving that she was willing to invest money in her own health and future.

Suzanne's newly won confidence helped her find better job opportunities. In 1972 she landed a minor role in a feature movie, George Lucas's *American Graffiti*. The film was a tremendous success, and even though Suzanne appeared in only one scene, her role as a beautiful blonde in a white Thunderbird was an image that audiences vividly remembered. The exposure brought her even more work: she was cast in a Clint Eastwood movie and began getting quite a bit of television work. Suzanne knew, however, that there wasn't enough of this kind of work in the San Francisco area. To really rise to the top in show business, she needed to move to Los Angeles, the center of the American film industry.

She also knew that she could not continue her relationship with Alan Hamel if he was not willing to commit to it. Hamel had divorced his wife, but he had never spoken to her about marriage or even about living together. Finally, she explained to him that unless he was seriously committed to staying involved with her, she would not continue seeing him. It was a very difficult decision for Suzanne. She loved Alan, but she knew that she had to respect herself first or else her love for him would turn to resentment and anger.

Suzanne was not the only member of her family who was trying to overcome her problems. Her sister, Maureen, had begun to realize that her drinking was destroying her life and those around her, and she began attending meetings of Alcoholics Anonymous. When Marion Mahoney learned about a support group for families of alcoholics, an organization known as Al-Anon, she began attending sessions as well. Soon,

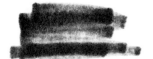

Marion's daughter-in-law—Danny's wife—began to accompany her. After some time, even Frank and Danny began attending Alcoholics Anonymous meetings, and Michael eventually accompanied them. Every member of the family had begun his or her own personal struggle to recover from the effects of the disease they had suffered from for many years.

Suzanne moved to Los Angeles in 1974. Alan had told her that he was ready to live with her, although he felt some guilt about living with Suzanne's son, Bruce, rather than with his own children. Alan and Suzanne struggled for some time to resolve the difficulties of combining their two families. Bruce resented the attention his mother paid Alan, and Alan's children resented Suzanne and blamed her for their parents' divorce. Over many years, they eventually resolved their problems.

In January 1977, Suzanne got the chance she'd dreamed of when she was cast as Chrissy Snow in *Three's Company,* a television sitcom about a single man sharing an apartment with two single women. The show brought Suzanne and her costars instant fame and quickly became one of the most popular shows on TV. The following year, Suzanne earned a People's Choice Award for her role in the series, and in 1979 she received a Golden Globe nomination for Best Actress in a Television Series.

Suzanne's career underwent great changes in 1980. She married Alan Hamel, who later became her business manager as well. Alan negotiated a two-year contract with the MGM Grand Hotel in Las Vegas, Nevada, for Suzanne to produce and perform in her own show. Her show was so successful that she took it on the night-club circuit. She also hosted her own CBS musical special. But just when it seemed as though her

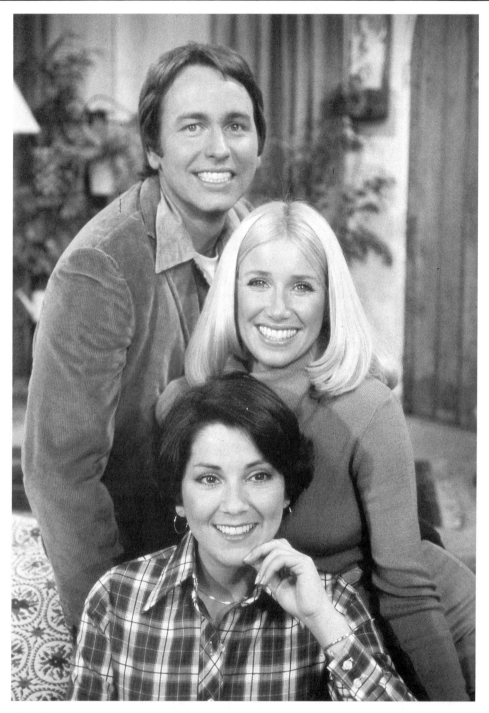

*The television sitcom* Three's Company *brought Suzanne Somers and her co-stars instant fame.*

career was taking off, she suffered a major setback. After she and Alan tried to negotiate for a better contract with *Three's Company* producers, the executives decided to replace her.

For several years after her departure from *Three's Company,* Suzanne dedicated herself to spending more time with her family. In 1984, however, the Las Vegas Hilton contacted Suzanne looking for a "headliner" to draw crowds to their establishment. The hotel offered her a six-month contract to perform regular shows there. Suzanne drew full houses during her entire run, and as a result her contract was extended to three years. Now with a steady job, Suzanne found time to begin writing a book about her childhood, which she called *Keeping Secrets.* The book landed on the *New York Times* best-seller list after it was published in 1988.

Not until four years later, during a trip to France for her stepson Stephen's wedding, did Suzanne first hear about the principles of a new diet program known as food combining. She heard about it from her stepson's in-laws when, after a wonderful meal at their home, she began picking and eating cherries from an orchard on the grounds. Stephen's father-in-law warned them not to eat the cherries after their meal, explaining later that fruit should be eaten on an empty stomach or else it might cause indigestion.

When Suzanne returned to the United States, she began researching food combining, and she tried several diets based on its principles. She discovered that most of them were too restrictive in one way or another: either they did not allow carbohydrates, or they allowed only limited proteins and fats. "My objective," she later explained, "was to find a way to eat healthy, nutritious, yet flavorful foods in substantial portions and still lose weight."

The plan Suzanne Somers devised is called "Somersizing," and she emphasizes that it is not strictly a "diet." Rather, she declares, it is "a weight-loss solution to the diet roller coaster . . . a whole new way of eating that will change your thinking about losing weight and gaining energy." Suzanne divides the eating plan, which can be categorized as a food-combining method, into two levels. Level One is for weight loss; Level Two is for maintenance once a desired weight has been achieved. She calls the three steps involved in level one "eliminate," "separate," and "combine."

Foods that are eliminated include sugars, alcohol, caffeine, and refined flour and other high-starch foods. The first three of these substances are high in calories but contain little nutrition. Instead, they pro-

*Suzanne has created dozens of delicious recipes for her cookbooks.*

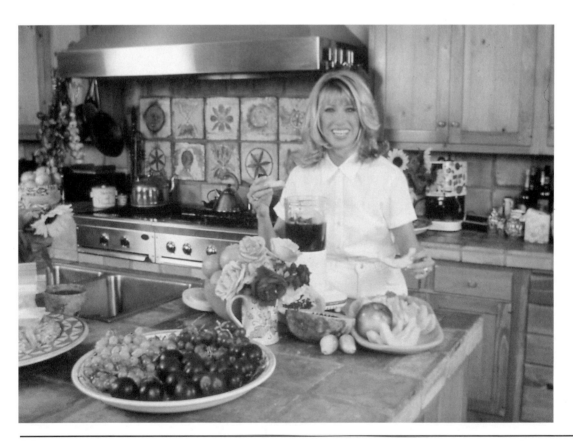

vide quick energy that the body will use instead of resorting to its fat reserves. The third substance, caffeine, is a stimulant, and it interferes with the metabolism and increases appetite, claims Suzanne.

Foods that have not been eliminated are then divided into carbohydrates, vegetables, proteins/fats, and fruits. These divisions make up in simplicity what they lack in scientific accuracy (since many fruits and vegetables also contain carbohydrates). The rules for combining these categories are not as straightforward, however: fruits are eaten by themselves and on an empty stomach. In practice, this usually means that fruit is consumed first thing in the morning, for breakfast. After eating fruit, one must wait half an hour before switching to either carbohydrates or proteins/fats. The dieter cannot consume fruit after eating any other category of food unless at least two hours have passed. Vegetables can be combined either with carbohydrates or proteins/fats, but carbohydrates and proteins/fats must never be eaten together at the same meal. Furthermore, Suzanne says that one must wait at least three hours between a carbohydrate meal and a protein/fat meal.

The theory here seems simple enough. It is difficult to digest different foods, particularly proteins and carbohydrates, at the same time, claim proponents of food-combining plans. This slower digestion process causes bloating and indigestion and promotes fat storage. Furthermore, the more complicated digestion process takes more energy and can cause lethargy. There is nothing to measure or count in such diet plans; no supplements are required, and very few foods must be eliminated. But in practice the program is more complicated. For example, carrots and bananas are both grouped as sugars, and therefore must be eliminated in the Level One, or weight-loss, part of the Somersizing plan. Also, only skim milk is allowed—even low-fat milk must be eliminated because it combines fat with carbohydrates.

The tricky part of practicing Somersizing or any other food-combining regime is finding out whether there are any fats at all in meals that include carbohydrates. This means, for instance, that you cannot use oil in salad dressing or pasta sauces, and that you cannot use mayonnaise or similar spreads on vegetarian sandwiches (there are no other kinds of sandwiches in the Somersizing plan, because you cannot combine carbohydrates with protein).

Suzanne Somers' most recent books, *Eat Great, Lose Weight* (1997) and *Get Skinny on Fabulous Food* (1999), are primarily cookbooks that include recipes based on the Somersizing method. It is clearly a weight-control method for those who love food and love to cook. Suzanne has gathered recipes from her travels around the world, and she uses fresh herbs from her own garden. The way meals are presented is also important to her. She loves fine linens and lace, beautiful table settings of china and old silver, and her book explores this as well. In a context of rich impressions and good company, she believes, meals become an emotional experience worth treasuring—and at the same time they promote a healthy and trim body.

# Chronology

1946  Born on October 16 in San Bruno, California

1963  Expelled from Catholic high school

1964  Graduates from public high school; enrolls at Lone Mountain College; marries Bruce Somers

1965  Son, Bruce, is born

1967  Divorces Bruce Somers and moves to Sausalito

1968  Meets Alan Hamel at KGO Studios in San Francisco

1970  Arrested for check fraud

1971  Son Bruce seriously injured when struck by car

1972  Appears in *American Graffiti*

1974  Moves to Los Angeles

1977  Cast as Chrissy Snow in the popular television sitcom *Three's Company*

1978  Wins People's Choice Award for Favorite Actress in a New Series

1979  Nominated for Golden Globe for Best Actress in a Television Series

1980  Marries Alan Hamel, who becomes her manager; loses role on *Three's Company*

1984  Begins starring in a Las Vegas Hilton stage show

1987  Begins filming television series *She's the Sheriff*

1988  Publishes autobiography, *Keeping Secrets*; begins a lecture tour

1991  Stars in TV sitcom *Step by Step;* son is married; stepson Stephen is married

1996  Publishes *Eat Great, Lose Weight*

1998  Publishes *After the Fall*

1999  Publishes *Get Skinny on Fabulous Food*

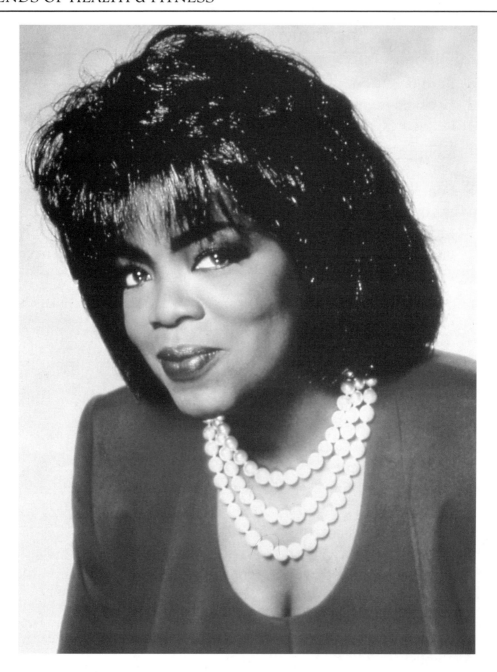

*Oprah Winfrey is one of the most famous and highly paid entertainers in the world.*

# CHAPTER THREE
## Oprah Winfrey

Oprah Winfrey is one of the wealthiest and most powerful women in the world. Practically every newsstand, it seems, features her face on at least one magazine cover. Millions of people tune in daily to her TV talk show, and she has received an Academy Award nomination for her acting skills. The books she recommends in her on-air book club immediately leap onto best-seller lists, and the causes she champions are guaranteed success. In 1998, *Forbes* magazine named Winfrey the fourth-highest paid entertainer in the world, with earnings of $125 million per year.

Oprah's amazing talent for putting others at ease has made her the most successful TV talk show host ever. Her ambition and determination to succeed have brought her scores of achievements. But for most of her life, Oprah Winfrey has suffered countless defeats in one regard—controlling her weight. At 5 feet 7 inches tall, she is of average height, but at one point she weighed 237 pounds. For much of her adult life, Oprah Winfrey felt desperately unhappy about herself because she had great difficulty not only shedding extra pounds but also keeping them off. Trying diet after diet, she often succeeded in losing great amounts of weight, but each time she would gain it all back—and sometimes she would even put on more weight. Each time, that is, until she finally faced the complex problems that were causing her weight gain.

Because Oprah Winfrey is constantly in the public eye, her weight problems are familiar to millions of her fans. Winfrey has bravely shared many of the details of her successes and failures, speaking honestly about the physical and emotional obstacles she encountered in her efforts to lose weight, achieve fitness, and live a healthier, more active life.

Oprah Winfrey was born on January 29, 1954, to Vernita Lee, a young unmarried girl who identified the father of her baby as Vernon Winfrey, a 20-year-old soldier who had returned to active duty. Vernita intended to give her daughter the Biblical name "Orpah," from the Book of Ruth, but in the official birth records of Kosciusko, Mississippi, where she was born, the second and third letters of the name were transposed, making her "Oprah" instead.

Soon after Oprah's birth, Vernita Lee headed north to find a better life, leaving her daughter with her own mother, Hattie Mae Lee, on an isolated pig farm for the first six years of her life. Hattie Mae knew that education provided the best hope for a black woman. As soon as Oprah could understand her, Hattie Mae began tutoring the child in reading, writing, and arithmetic; by the time Oprah was three years old, she could read on her own. She also displayed a natural talent for reciting, and she performed several times at her grandmother's Baptist church. The adults in the congregation greatly admired little Oprah, but the other children envied her because of her favored status. "All the kids hated me, all through school," Oprah remembers, "but the teachers loved me."

By the time Oprah began attending kindergarten, her teacher realized that she had already advanced beyond the other children, and she moved her to first grade. Shunned by the older children, Oprah turned to reading books and spending time with the farm animals for comfort. Whenever she disobeyed her grandmother, she could count on a whipping. It was a lonely and hard life for a little girl, but one that laid a foundation of discipline and hard work.

In 1960, when Oprah was six years old, Vernita sent for her to come to Milwaukee, Wisconsin, where she had settled. Vernita had had another child by then—Oprah's half-sister, Patricia—but she still had not married. She and the two little girls lived in a one-room boarding house in a run-down section of Milwaukee. Vernita worked as a maid in the suburbs, so she had to leave the boarding house very early each morning to get to work, and she returned late each night. The children didn't see much of their mother.

Vernita had hoped to marry Patricia's father, but the man drifted off. Exhausted from working and caring for her two children, Vernita contacted Vernon Winfrey to see whether he could take in Oprah. By this time, Vernon was living in Nashville, Tennessee, and married to another woman, Zelma, but the couple did not have children and were glad to have Oprah come to live with them. Oprah began third grade in Nashville.

Zelma was a strict disciplinarian, just as Oprah's grandmother was, and she was every bit as determined to see that Oprah received a solid education. In addition to school work, Zelma demanded that Oprah read a book every week—and write a report about it. Seven-year-old Oprah was still showing talent in other ways as well: she earned a $500 reward for delivering a speech to a church group. After all her hard work during the school year, Oprah was glad to see summer arrive so she could take some time off and visit her mother again.

Oprah had adjusted well to living with her father and his wife, so she was disappointed when she learned that her mother wanted her to stay in Milwaukee. Vernita had met another man whom she intended to marry, and she wanted her whole family to live together. The man didn't stay long, however, and after he left Vernita gave birth to a third child, named Jeffrey. Oprah missed her father and Zelma and the security of their Nashville home. Her father was angry when Oprah was not returned to them. He knew that Oprah was better off with him, but he could do nothing about the situation.

The crowded two-bedroom apartment in which Vernita and her children lived was also home to a new boyfriend of hers, as well as other relatives who came and went regularly. Only years later, when Oprah was already a popular talk-show host, would she admit that during this time she was sexually abused by several men—first, a 14-year-old cousin who raped her, and later others. She said, "I didn't tell anybody about it because I thought I would be blamed for it. I remember blaming myself for it, thinking something must be wrong with me."

Oprah's troubles at school only added to the terror of being abused at home. Although she excelled academically despite her home life, she continued to be unpopular with her classmates. On several occasions, some of them threatened to beat her up. Finally, one of her teachers noticed the girl's predicament and recommended her for a special scholarship program called Upward Bound, which helped minority students get into private (often all-white) schools, where they would receive better educations. In 1968, when Oprah was 14, she received a full scholarship to Nicolet High School in the upper-class, predominantly white suburb of Fox Lake. The school was 20 miles and three bus transfers from the ghetto where Oprah lived with her mother and half-sister. "I was feeling a sense of anguish, because living with my mother in Milwaukee, I was in a situation where I was the only black kid, and I mean the only one, in a school of two thousand upper-middle-class suburban Jewish kids," Oprah has said of that time in her life. "I would take the bus in the morning to school with the maids who worked in their homes. The life that I saw those children lead was so totally different from what I went home to."

Torn by guilt and still suffering from the psychological effects of being sexually abused, Oprah began to rebel. She ran away from home several times, and she would chase after boys and bring them back to the apartment to have sex. On one occasion, she stayed away from home for a week, and when she ran out of money she called the family minister so she wouldn't have to face her mother's anger alone. But as far as her mother was concerned, Oprah had gone too far. Her mother took her to a home for wayward girls, where she intended to have her committed. Fortunately, the institution had no room for Oprah, and its supervisor told Vernita to bring her daughter back in two weeks. Instead, Vernita decided to call Vernon, who drove to Milwaukee and took his daughter back to Nashville.

Once Oprah was back with them, Zelma realized that her step-daughter had become pregnant. But Oprah miscarried, and finally she poured out the story of all the men with whom she had had sex. Vernon and Zelma were stunned. The girl in front of them was very different from the nine-year-old who had left them five years earlier, in 1963. She wore short tight skirts, halter tops, and heavy makeup, and she had a smart mouth and a lot of pent-up anger and shame. But not for long.

Vernon and Zelma laid down the law for Oprah. They demanded that she change her behavior and that she bring home high grades from school. Oprah was smart enough to realize that she had a chance to turn her life around. "I got sent to live with my father so that my father could straighten me out, and that he did," she remembers. The academic rules that Vernon and Zelma expected Oprah to follow included making straight *As* and doing lots of extra reading. The reading projects exposed the troubled girl to a world of new authors, including African-American writers like Alice Walker and Maya Angelou. Oprah felt particularly drawn to Angelou's autobiographical book, *I Know Why the Caged Bird Sings*, which describes a childhood that in many ways was similar to Oprah's—Angelou herself was shuttled from home to home as a child, and she suffered a traumatic rape that caused her to stop speaking for several years. The story was so like Oprah's own experiences that, years later, she met Angelou and developed a close friendship with the author.

Oprah was expected to excel in school not only for her own sake, but because she was one of the first black students admitted to East Nashville High School. She was active in drama classes, and she was elected student council president. Before long, there was no trace of the wild, rebellious, and promiscuous girl from Milwaukee in this conservatively dressed, obedient Nashville teenager. When Oprah was 17, she represented East Nashville High at a White House Conference on Youth in Colorado, and she participated in a speaking competition. She was also giving recitations in Nashville, where she was asked to appear before church and civic groups several times a month. In her senior year, Oprah also received other honors that she would never have imagined she could earn: classmates voted her "Most Popular Girl," and after a local radio station sponsored her in a Miss Fire Prevention competition, she became the first black in Nashville to win the contest. Although Vernon did not completely approve, Oprah also entered other beauty contests—and her father was pleased when she won a four-year scholarship to Tennessee State University (TSU) as a prize in one of the contests.

In 1971, while she was still a senior in high school, Oprah took a part-time job broadcasting for radio station WVOL in Nashville. She was responsible for delivering the news reports on weekends and after school. After she began attending TSU, she continued working at the station, and in 1973 she was offered a job on television. Station WTVF-TV was looking for minority employees, and they offered Oprah a position as an on-air newscaster.

Oprah knew that her father would disapprove of her dropping out of college to take the position, but a drama teacher helped her explain to Vernon that one of the reasons for earning a college education was to enable Oprah to get opportunities like the one she had already been offered. So at 19 years old, Oprah Winfrey left TSU and became the first female and the first black newscaster in Nashville.

Oprah worked at WTVF for three years. At 22 years old, she was still living with Vernon and Zelma, and she began to feel as though she needed a change. She was grateful for all her father and stepmother had done, but she believed it was time to strike out on her own. "My father saved my life at a time when I needed to be saved," she said. "He turned my life around by insisting I be more than I was and by believing I could be more. His love of learning showed me the way." So when Oprah was offered a position at WJZ-TV in Baltimore, Maryland, she took it.

Oprah moved to Baltimore in the summer of 1976. She has described her experiences during her first year with WJZ-TV as the darkest time of her career. The station's news director, who had hired Oprah for her warm, relaxed style, suddenly decided he didn't like it after all. Her co-anchor on the evening news program disliked working with her. She was criticized for nearly everything, from the way she looked and dressed to her habit of developing an emotional bond with the people she interviewed. The station hired a well-known dressmaker to change Oprah's style, and they sent her to an expensive French beauty salon for a makeover. The hair treatment she received there caused all of her hair to fall out, and she was forced to wear scarves on the air to cover her head while it grew back.

During this bleak period, Oprah started turning to food for consolation. Every night after her newscast, she would stop at the food booths in the shopping mall across the street from her apartment and pick up rich, comforting foods. By the fall of 1976 she had gained 10 pounds, and in an effort to lose the weight she went to her first diet doctor, who put her on a low-calorie diet— and also gave her diet pills. The pills, she said, "made me as crazy as a betsy bug! I stopped taking them after about a week." She did lose the 10 pounds, but by the end of the year she had gained it back.

Finally, more than a year after she arrived in Baltimore, her career took a turn for the better. In the fall of 1978, she managed to launch her own local talk show. But though the show was a great success, Oprah's attempt to stay slim had failed. As she continued gaining weight, she tried every diet she could find, from programs that required eating only protein and fats to all-carbohydrate diets. Oprah remembers, "In those days, I could lose an average of ten pounds in two weeks. . . . I thought I'd do better with a group. So I joined Weight Watchers, followed by Diet Workshop and Diet Center, and later Nutri-Systems. Every one of these worked—for a while." After eight years in Baltimore, Oprah Winfrey weighed 172 pounds.

In 1984, Oprah heard of a talk-show host position opening up in Chicago, Illinois, but she didn't think she had a chance of getting the job. She decided to go on an interview anyway. Once in the room with the head of the Chicago station, she came right to the point. "Well, you know, I'm overweight and black," she told him. "Yeah," he said, "I can see. I'm looking at you. No one in here is going to complain about that. And as for being black, it wouldn't matter to me what color you were; I think you have a gift and I'd like you to share it with this television station."

Delighted at the reception she received, Oprah took the job and moved to Chicago in December 1983 to host *A.M. Chicago* (which in 1985 became *The Oprah Winfrey Show*.) Oprah loved Chicago—and Chicago loved Oprah. Her success was immediate: within four weeks the show leapt in the ratings from last in its time period to first, and within just 12 weeks twice as many viewers were watching Oprah as were watching Phil Donahue, the previously unchallenged champion of Chicago talk television.

But as her success grew, Oprah continued to put on weight. By the end of her first year in Chicago, she had gained another 28 pounds and weighed 202. Over the next four years, she would gain another 16 pounds. The knowledge that she needed to take action to control her weight and her health hit her with force while she was attending a boxing match one evening, where the announcer introduced Mike Tyson, who weighed in at 218 pounds. She thought, "I weigh as much as the heavyweight champion of the world," and she left that night determined to do something about her problem.

All the while, Oprah was succeeding dramatically in her career. She began appearing on national television, including a guest appearance on the *Tonight Show*. In 1985 she landed a role as Sofia in Steven Spielberg's film *The Color Purple*, based on Alice Walker's novel of the same name, a longtime favorite book of Oprah's. It was a great honor for her to appear in the movie, which was a tremendous success: it received 11 Academy Award nominations, including one for Oprah as Best Supporting Actress.

Oprah had a special gown designed for the Oscars ceremony in February 1986. She had been gaining weight, but the designer had come to her hotel suite and fitted the gown to her figure. When it was delivered just before the ceremony, however, Oprah couldn't get into it. In desperation, she decided to lie on the floor and have her friends pull it up around her. On the way to the awards ceremony, she couldn't sit down in the tight gown, so she again had to lie down—on the floor of the limousine. She didn't even want to win an Oscar because she was afraid the seams of the dress would split if she had to walk up the stage steps to accept the award. The embarrassment and shame she experienced that night would stay with her for a long time, and make her even more determined to try to control her weight for good.

That year was one of her great career successes, however. Oprah appeared in another film, based on Richard Wright's novel *Native Son*. *The Oprah Winfrey Show* went into syndication, meaning that it would be broadcast from television stations all over the country (by the King Syndicate, in which Oprah owned stock). In 1986 she also launched her own production company, Harpo Productions, which allowed her to produce her own films and television programs. And in her personal life, she began dating Stedman Graham, a public relations executive with whom Oprah would finally develop a secure and loving relationship.

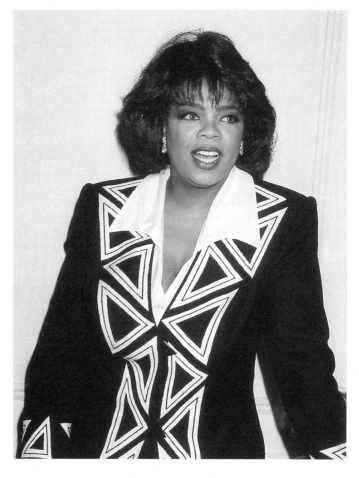

*Oprah often succeeded in losing large amounts of weight, but each time she would gain it back.*

In 1988 Oprah, who was still struggling to control her weight, heard about a weight-loss program called Optifast, a regime that included fasting and taking liquid nutritional supplements. She decided to try it, and for four months, beginning in July, she stayed on the program. By fall, she had lost 67 pounds and fit into a size 10 dress. Oprah had shared these months of following the medically supervised diet with her talk-show

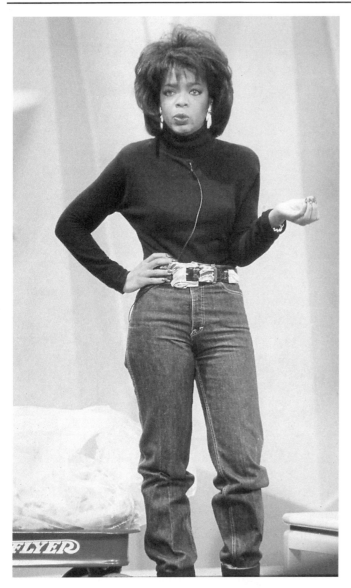

*Oprah in size 10 jeans after losing 67 pounds on the Optifast diet.*

audience, and on November 15, 1988, she opened the program by pulling a wagon onto the stage that was loaded with 67 pounds of animal fat—a vivid representation of the amount of weight she had lost while on the Optifast diet. Skeptics believed that she would gain the weight back, but Oprah disagreed. She was sure that she had won the battle to stay slim and that her war against fat was over.

For the next five years, however, Oprah's nightmare of weight loss and gain continued. Two weeks after her triumphant appearance with the wagon of animal fat, Oprah had gained five pounds; a year later she had gained 15 additional pounds; two years later she again weighed more than 200 pounds. In 1992, Oprah attended the Daytime Emmy Awards ceremony weighing more than she ever had before—237 pounds. "Outwardly, I was becoming more popular and successful," she says. "Inside, the burden of weight was always there. It never left me."

She decided to make another concerted effort to take off the excess weight and keep it off. She had heard of a new spa that was opening in Colorado and went there for a three-week stay. There she met Bob Greene, a personal trainer who would help her understand why she was having so much difficulty controlling her weight, and who would provide her with the program that would finally put her on the path to health and fitness. Oprah enjoyed working with him so much that in early 1993 she asked him to come to Chicago to help her stick to her new fitness regime. He told her, "I'm only going to work with you if you're willing to be here every day without fail, no excuses."

"I really liked Bob's approach," Oprah says. "There was nothing bullying or judgmental about it. He was very matter-of-fact and very confident. . . . There was no secret. 'It's all physics,' he said. I believed him. So I looked him straight in the eye and said, 'Okay, no problem.'" Bob Greene taught Oprah his 10 steps for weight loss and fitness, and the physiological reasons why each one was necessary:

1. Exercise aerobically in the morning five to seven days each week.
2. Exercise "in the zone" (Greene sets levels of intensity to measure workouts; "in the zone" means at a high level of intensity).
3. Exercise for 20 to 60 minutes each session.
4. Eat a low-fat, balanced diet.
5. Eat three meals and two snacks each day.
6. Limit or eliminate alcohol consumption.
7. Stop eating two to three hours before bedtime.
8. Drink six to eight glasses of water each day.
9. Have at least two servings of fruit and three servings of vegetables daily.
10. Renew your commitment to healthy living each day.

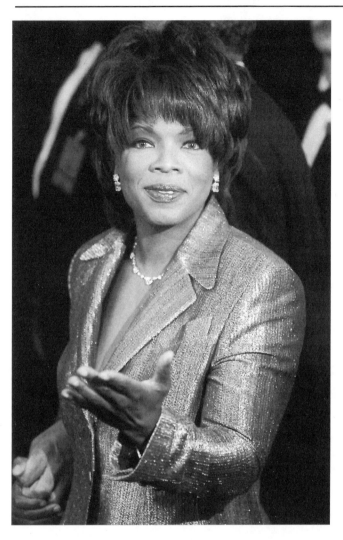

*In 1996, Oprah's book on fitness reached the top of the best-seller list.*

Once Oprah had more information about how the human body works—and once she realized how much better she felt while following Greene's program—she felt ready to take complete responsibility for her weight and her health.

The first three steps of Bob Greene's program deal with exercise, and he emphasizes that they are important because they affect the metabolism. When a person exercises correctly—at the right time of day, consistently, with enough intensity, and long enough during each session—the metabolic rate (the rate at which the body "burns" fat) will increase. Greene believes that morning hours are the best time to exercise, because it increases one's metabolism for the remainder of the day. The "zone" he refers to is determined by the individual's heart rate—the exercise should be intense enough to increase that rate to 70 or 80 percent of its maximum capacity. Bob Greene found that a level of exercise that placed Oprah in the proper zone would be too low for him—so after working out with her, he would have to continue his own workout at a higher intensity to satisfy his personal requirements. The amount of time a person needs to spend in his or her proper zone of intensity also varies. Some can burn fat with 20 minutes of exercise each day; others require 60 minutes to reach the same point. Oprah discovered that she has to exercise "in her zone" for at least 45 to 50 minutes daily to control her weight.

Even when Oprah was training to run in a marathon—which she did in 1994 to celebrate her 40th birthday—she found that she gradually gained some weight, despite her schedule of running 15 or 20 miles daily. Why? Because running for such long distances did not allow her to maintain the rapid pace necessary to sustain her proper zone. But because she was determined to run the marathon, she was willing to make the sacrifice of gaining three or four pounds.

The kind of aerobic exercise a person chooses to perform doesn't matter, says Greene, as long as it elevates the heart rate to a consistent level and keeps it there for the duration of the session. Of course, it makes sense to find a routine that is enjoyable, or at least fairly easy to stick with. Greene suggests finding one main form of exercise and then alternating with one or two others to add variety to your daily workout. Oprah's first choice was jogging or running, but on occasion she would substitute with swimming or rowing.

Oprah's full schedule required that she wake up an hour earlier each morning to exercise. "I'm proud to say that I've done it almost every day, without fail," she has said. "I no longer even vacation in a place where I can't find a treadmill or a road I can walk or jog on. And on vacation it's the first thing I do when I wake up. I get at least 40 minutes out of the way so I can more fully enjoy the rest of my day."

Some of the steps Greene used to help regulate Oprah's diet were not entirely new to her. She already

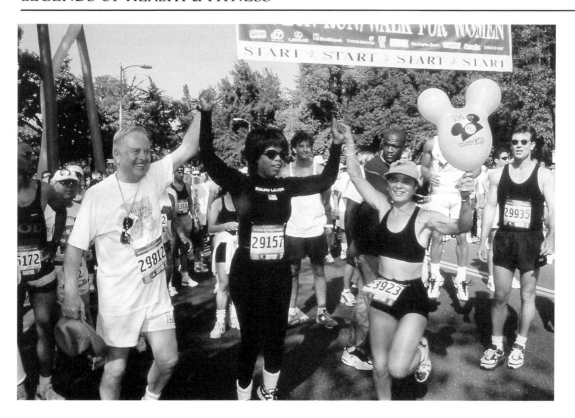

*Oprah with Mayor Riordan in the Revlon Charity Race for Women in May of 1997.*

had a cook, Rosie Daley, who specialized in preparing low-fat meals. But that wasn't enough. "For me, just reducing fat wasn't enough to lose the excess pounds," Oprah has said. "For two years before I met Bob I ate only low-fat meals and snacks. Not only did I not lose weight, I gained. Partly because I never learned when to stop eating. I was a compulsive emotional eater." Becoming more aware of when and why she ate was an important step in Oprah's education. Under Greene's guidance, she realized that she hardly ever ate simply because she felt hungry. Instead, she ate when she was under stress—and with her busy schedule that meant most of the time—and at regularly scheduled meal times, which usually were social occasions that included staff and friends. She hadn't learned to listen to the actual demands of her body. One of Bob's first suggestions was that she not eat unless she was truly hungry. It was difficult, but Oprah finally learned that she needed to follow the physical demands of her own body instead of catering to her emotions.

Oprah also learned that *when* she ate was important. Instead of eating a large dinner every evening, she began consuming the same amount of food in smaller meals spread throughout the day. Breakfast, lunch, and dinner were supplemented with two light snacks. Oprah observed, "I've learned that when I eat smaller meals throughout the day, I'm less hungry and I get the added benefit of keeping the flame under that metabolism of mine. When you eat this way you never get that stuffed, let-me-roll-onto-the-sofa, Thanksgiving feeling. You're burning calories more efficiently." Greene also stressed that she should avoid eating within two to three hours of going to bed, because the metabolism slows when one is asleep.

Some of the changes Bob suggested turned out to be a delight for Oprah. She had never really experimented with different fruits and vegetables because she considered them boring. But since two servings of fruit and three servings of vegetables became a requirement, she says, "I've expanded my awareness and developed some new favorites." Other changes were more difficult. She doesn't like drinking water, even though she is supposed to drink six to eight glasses each day. "I've tried water plain out of the tap, bottled sparkling [water], bottled [water] without carbonation. With a slice of lime, a slice of lemon, or an orange wedge," Oprah says, "I've had it right out of the bottle, in small glasses, large glasses, plain glasses, and fancy glasses. And the bottom line is, I still don't like it." But Oprah forces herself to drink at least six glasses a day because she now understands how it helps her body.

Bob Greene explained that drinking plenty of water is essential to weight control for several reasons. It helps the digestive and metabolic systems to work at top efficiency, and it helps diminish one's appetite. Sometimes your body may seem to be telling you that it is hungry when actually it needs water, so it's important to pay attention to such "cues." Another important fact is that lean muscle requires water. As fat is lost and lean muscle gained, more water is required.

Bob Greene's program finally enabled Oprah Winfrey to change her life and stop the roller-coaster weight gain and loss. Her story is outlined in *Make the Connection,* which Winfrey and Greene coauthored in 1996. Oprah has continued to maintain a fairly consistent weight, and five years after she finally attained her goal of weighing 150 pounds, she is fit and healthy and has plenty of energy to get her through her busy days. Though Oprah's weight may still fluctuate slightly, she now knows that she can make decisions about her own fitness based on solid facts about what her body requires. With her very slow metabolism, she may find it more efficient to carry a little more weight than she'd like instead of struggling in longer, more strenuous exercise sessions. Either way, it is finally Oprah Winfrey's decision. She is no longer a victim of weight gain—knowledge has put her in control of her own body.

# Chronology

1954  Born on January 29 in Kosciusko, Mississippi

1968  Receives a full scholarship to Nicolet High School

1971  Represents East Nashville High at a White House Conference on Youth; is voted Most Popular Girl in high school; wins title of Miss Fire Prevention; begins working for radio station WVOL

1973  Becomes first female and first black TV newscaster in Nashville on TV station WTVF

1976  Moves to Baltimore, Maryland, to work as newscaster for WJZ-TV

1983  Moves to Chicago to host *A.M. Chicago*

1985  *A.M. Chicago* is renamed *The Oprah Winfrey Show;* is cast as Sofia in Spielberg's *The Color Purple*

1986  Nominated for a Best Supporting Actress Oscar for her role in *The Color Purple;* stars in *Native Son;* establishes Harpo Productions

1988  Loses 67 pounds on Optifast program

1992  Wins Daytime Emmy Award, but weighs 237 pounds

1993  Invites Bob Greene to Chicago as her personal trainer

1994  Completes a marathon to celebrate her 40th birthday; wins Daytime Emmys for Best Show and Best Host

1996  Coauthors *Make the Connection* with Bob Greene

1998  Produces and stars in *Toni Morrison's Beloved;* is named fourth-highest paid entertainer by *Forbes* magazine

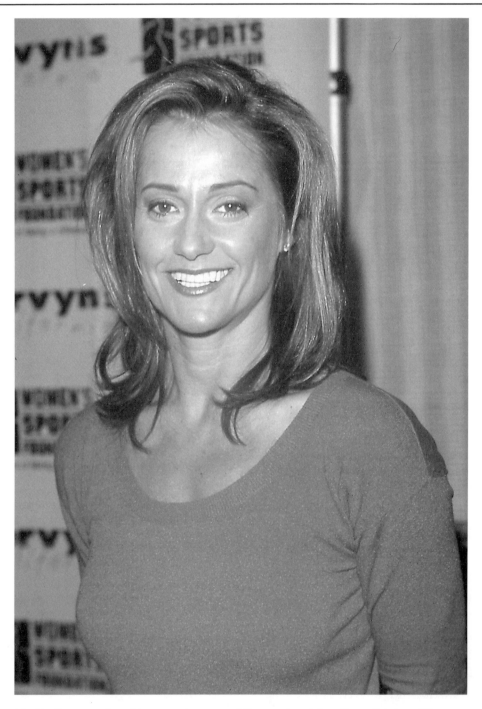

*Nadia Comaneci's achievement as one of the most outstanding athletes of the twentieth century is based on remarkable self-discipline.*

# CHAPTER FOUR
# Nadia Comaneci

**N**adia Comaneci is widely agreed to be one of the most outstanding athletes of the twentieth century. This young gymnast accomplished feats that were believed to be impossible—such as receiving perfect scores in Olympic and other international competitions—not just once, but consistently in her competitive career. Nadia is one of 25 members of the World Sports Academy for Laureus Sports Awards Winners, and in 1999 she was voted one of the 25 Oustanding Sports People of the Century by the International Association of Sports Writers. She also was selected as one of the top 100 athletes of the century in a poll by *Sports Illustrated*, finishing at number nine.

Nadia Comaneci's life has been full of excitement, adventure, and accomplishments. And all of these have been based on remarkable motivation and self-discipline. To achieve what she has achieved, she had to master all aspects of self-control. She had to control her body, not only in the difficult physical movements she had to master, but also in controlling her weight and her energy so that she would have enough endurance for the demanding routines she had to perform. On those few occasions when she slipped, when she fell from the bars or the balance beam, or when she lost control of her weight and excess pounds threatened her career, she had the courage and the will to start again. And she had the determination to succeed again.

Nadia was born on November 12, 1961, in the town of Onesti, Romania, which is located in the foothills of the Carpathian Mountains. Before a program of industrialization was instituted by the Communist Party of Romania, Onesti had been a small foresting village in the beautiful province of Moldavia. It was still a magical place of natural beauty and kind, friendly people during the years Nadia was growing up. Her father was a mechanic who serviced the huge foresting tractors and machinery used in the area, and her mother worked in a hospital.

Even when she was an infant, Nadia's curiosity and her love for movement and adventure kept her parents constantly on guard. When she was two years old she pulled down the family Christmas tree trying to get at one of the delicious candies that were hanging on it. As her father pulled her out of the broken pine branches, he laughed to see that she was still clutching the sweet she had been determined to grab. Since then, Nadia says, she has managed to get to the sweets without so much destruction.

Growing up, one of Nadia's favorite activities was climbing the many trees that lined the streets of Onesti. When she visited her grandparents' home across the river, she headed straight for the orchard and climbed the fruit trees. One afternoon after she had spent hours in the top of a plum tree, her grandmother tried to coax her down with home-made cookies, but even for the sweets she loved, Nadia wouldn't come down. Her grandmother went off shaking her head, saying, "She's a strange little thing." With all of her relatives living close by in Onesti, and lots of cousins to play with, Nadia never felt the lack of warm family affection.

When she was three years old, Nadia began kindergarten. Her mother and father hoped that the activities at the school would help burn some of little Nadia's seemingly boundless energy. Her favorite time came when the children were taught an elementary form of gymnastics by one of the teachers. She waited each week for gym time to come around. Her favorite activities were turning cartwheels and doing acrobatics, and after that she liked playing soccer with the boys. When she proved she was as good as they were, they let her join in their games.

Meanwhile, the man who was to become one of the most significant people in Nadia Comaneci's life had started a gymnastics school in the small town of Vulcan. Bela Karolyi, a man who has coached more national and world title holders and Olympic medalists in gymnastics than anyone else in the world, and his wife Marta Eross started their gymnastics school with the aim to produce world-class gymnasts by recruiting very young girls with special talent. Bela and Marta had started their school in 1963, the year they were married, after meeting as gymnasts at the Physical Education University in Bucharest. Their plan worked so well that by 1968 Bela was the Romanian Olympic gymnastics coach.

According to Bela Karolyi's account, he was visiting the kindergarten in the town of Onesti, scouting for talent for the National Junior Team, when he saw two little girls playing in the courtyard during recreation period. The girls were running and jumping around, pretending to be gymnasts. Just then the bell rang and the two girls ran inside with all of the other children.

He said he knew he would not leave that school until he found those girls again. He went through all of the kindergarten rooms twice without seeing them, so the third time through he asked the classes, "Who loves gymnastics?" In one class two little girls jumped up shouting, "We do! We do!"

One of those little girls was Nadia Comaneci. (The other became a successful ballerina.) Nadia's parents, who were still eager to find healthy uses for their daughter's excess energy, gladly consented to her being recruited for gymnastics school. Her coach observed later, "Nadia would have made something of herself, even if not for gymnastics. She is intelligent; she is dedicated and strong of spirit. She had a good physique, but that wasn't as important as her fire and enthusiasm."

The new gymnastics school was just a ten-minute walk from her home, and Nadia soon became accustomed to the routine. Gymnastics training was held from eight to noon every morning, with academic lessons in the afternoons. Frequently, especially when there were competitions coming up, there would be additional coaching in the gym in the evening. On top of that there was homework to do. Her meals were carefully regulated and she had lunch and her evening meal with the other students so her diet could be watched and changed according to the demands of the training. In addition to the coaches, there was a complete staff, including doctors, physiotherapists, nutritionists, choreographers, and musicians, to assist the girls with their training. Romania, like the other communist countries of Eastern Europe at that time, gave strong financial support to developing winning athletes.

In 1969, when she was seven years old, Nadia entered the Romanian National Junior Championships, her first official competition. She finished in 13th place, which actually was not bad for the youngest entry in the large field of gymnasts. Bela Karolyi, however, gave her a little Eskimo doll he had gotten in Canada and told her that the doll should remind her to never finish 13th again. It not only served that purpose, but became the first of a collection that would eventually include more than 200 dolls from all over the world.

Nadia, who by then had a little brother, Adrian, six years younger than she was, spent many evenings away from her family. She would stay at the gymnastics school dormitory so that she could practice late and start again early in the morning. The next year, 1970, her determination paid off when she won the Junior Championship. (She continued to carry the Eskimo doll with her to every competition.) In 1971 she won the Romanian all-around title for her age group. In 1972 she entered her first international competition, the Olympic Hopefuls meet which brought together gymnasts from all of the communist bloc countries of eastern Europe. Despite stiff competition, Nadia took three gold medals, and in the two following years she won the all-around title.

Of course the news about Nadia began to spread, particularly as she competed against the great Russian women gymnasts such as Olga Korbut, Nellie Kim, and Ludmilla Tourischeva. In 1975, Skien, Norway, was the location of the European Championships. This was the year that Nadia Comaneci became eligible to enter the senior international competition for the first time. The experts all believed that the contest would be between the Russians and the East German gymnasts, but it didn't turn out that way. On the first day Nadia won the overall four-event competition, and on the second

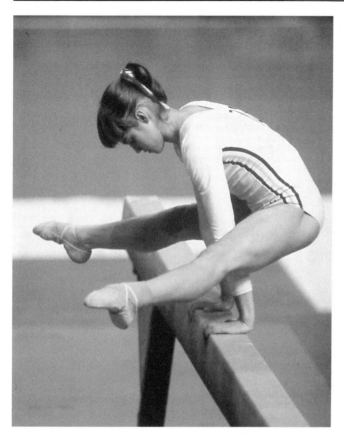

*Nadia earned a perfect score on the balance beam in the 1976 Montreal Olympics.*

day she won gold medals in vaulting, the uneven bars, and the balance beam. She took the silver medal in the floor exercises behind the Soviet Union's Nelli Kim.

A reporter described Nadia in Skien as "a thirteen-year-old fragile-looking child," and said that she "stunned the judges as well as the crowd not only with double somersaults and twists but also with an uncommon consistency and stability even in her most difficult moves." Nadia's confidence, and her strength that seemed impossible for so small a body, had everyone in the sports world talking.

People in America got to see Nadia Comaneci for the first time in the pre-Montreal Olympic qualifying events at Tucson, Albuquerque, San Francisco, Denver, and Toronto. Nadia surprised everyone by earning perfect scores in many of the events, something that the experts had thought was impossible. But Nadia, who had never been to the United States before, was more impressed with Disneyland than with her own performance.

After the preliminary events and qualifying meets for the Olympics, Nadia entered the American Cup competition in Madison Square Garden in New York City. In this event, one male and one female gymnast represent each of the participating nations. The two winners of the event, held in March of 1976, were 14-year-old

Nadia Comaneci of Romania and 18-year-old Bart Conner of the United States. As the two stood together with their big silver cups, a photographer said to Conner, "Why don't you lean down and give her a little kiss?" He did, although neither of them had any idea that 20 years later they would be married. "I wasn't interested in boys at that particular time," Nadia admitted later.

Four months after that kiss from Bart Conner in New York came the event that changed Nadia's life: the 1976 Montreal Olympic Games. As far as Nadia and the other girls on the Romanian Gymnastics Team were concerned, the tournament was not particularly unusual. What they did at Montreal was the result of years and years of discipline and practice, and then more discipline and more practice. But to the rest of the world, the audience in Montreal and the millions watching on television, Nadia's performance at the 1976 Olympics seemed miraculous, and the whole world went wild over this tiny 14-year-old from Romania.

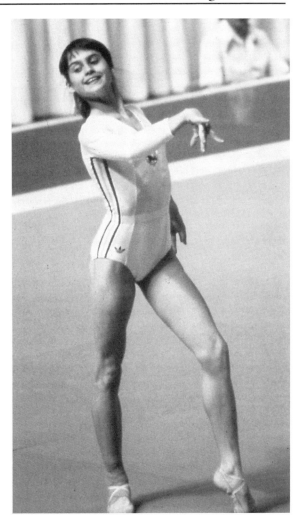

*Nadia won the gold medal as overall champion in the 1976 Olympics in Montreal.*

Nadia Comaneci became the first gymnast in Olympic history to earn a perfect score of 10 points in Olympic competition—and she did it not once but seven times! The newspapers called her "Little Miss Perfect," and for a week she was the most famous human being on earth, with her picture on the covers of *Time*,

*Newsweek,* and *Sports Illustrated* magazines. After she had won the gold medal as overall champion, Nadia said, "What I had achieved only began to sink in as I climbed the victory rostrum and, with the gold medal around my neck, watched the Romanian flag rise majestically to the sound of our National Anthem."

The girl who had stunned the world with her complete fearlessness and confidence on the balance beam and the bars was a little frightened by the frantic efforts of the crowds of newspapermen and photographers. Everywhere she went she was surrounded by microphones and questions, flashbulbs, people wanting her autograph, a frenzied mob trying to get close to her. Finally her coaches and the Olympic Committee agreed that it would be best if the Romanian team were allowed to return home early, without waiting for the closing ceremony.

Back in Romania the team received a hero's welcome and was honored at the Palace of Sport and Culture in Bucharest. Nadia was given another gold medal, this one as Hero of Socialist Labor by the President of Romania. Then the team left for a long and well-deserved summer holiday at a private beach on the coast of the Black Sea. After that it was back to the routine of training, although with the added duties of meeting dignitaries and enduring a certain amount of celebrity treatment.

Even though Nadia was back in training, however, nothing was the same as it had been before her dramatic victory at the Montreal Olympics. The drastic changes that occurred in the next two years affected just about every area of her life.

The most unsettling and disturbing change was the normal process of growing up, of changing from being a girl to being a woman. Nadia was late in experiencing the changes that come with puberty, a fact that caused some western observers to accuse the doctors and coaches of gymnasts in the communist countries of giving their young athletes drugs that retarded their natural development. Nadia and others insist that this is not so. Nadia says that it is perfectly normal for young women athletes to be late developers because their restricted diets and intense workouts cause less energy to be available for the body's development.

But whatever the reason for the late development, which did not begin until after she was 14 years old, in the years between 1976 and 1978 Nadia changed from a girl into a young woman. Along with the other physical changes, becoming taller and developing breasts and more rounded hips, she began gaining weight alarmingly. It took every bit of her will power to stick to the very restricted diet, primarily protein with fresh vegetables, that was required to keep her weight under control.

Along with her development from child to adult, came the necessity for more control over the decisions affecting her life and her career. Unfortunately, Bela Karolyi was not able to understand this. For 10 years this strong-willed, powerful man had been like a father to Nadia and the other young gymnnasts he coached to international fame. And like some other fathers, he was unable to see that when his "little ones," as he called them, were no longer little, he would have to allow them more freedom to make their own decisions. The brilliant, obstinant man and the brilliant, obstinant young woman were bound to have difficulties, and they did.

From details of her training routine to details of her performance routines, it seemed as though they were fighting about everything. Nadia objected to having every move she made supervised as though she were still a child. She wanted some time each week to relax, go to a movie with friends, or to a disco. Her coach wanted to continue to supervise her as though she were a child. Nadia wanted to make her own decisions about her competition routines. She felt that the little-girl flourishes and coy movements that Bela Karolyi insisted on were no longer appropriate for her rapidly developing body. Before long their battles were so explosive, and so disruptive to the Romanian team, that Nadia was assigned to a new coach, and her training location changed to the 23rd of August Sports Arena in Bucharest.

Changes were occurring in Nadia's family, too. Her parents had been having more and more difficulties, and under the stress of their disagreements her father had begun drinking heavily. Finally they divorced, and even though Nadia loved both of them very much, she felt that it was for the best. After they had separated her father stopped drinking and her mother seemed much happier with her new independence. Nadia and her mother and brother Adrian moved into a nice house in Bucharest only a short distance from the gym where she worked out.

Understandably, as she became a young woman with more freedom, and living in the big city instead of the small town of Onesti, Nadia rapidly developed an interest in clothes and cosmetics, things she had barely noticed before. She later admitted that for a while she overdressed and wore far too much make-up. "It took a while," she said, "before I realized that make up is supposed to enhance good features, not dominate them."

The newspapers in the western countries, still desperate for stories about "Little Miss Perfect" whether the stories were true or not, declared that Nadia was finished, that she was no longer motivated to compete, that she had attempted suicide after a disastrous love affair, and many other fanciful and completely unfounded tales. Nadia was in most cases completely unaware of what was being said about her, at least until long after the stories had been circulated. And even when she did find out, there was no way that she could demand that corrections be made. The only thing that she could do was what she did: she proved them wrong with the continued excellence of her performances and her gymnastic victories.

In her autobiography, *Nadia*, which was written before she was 20 years old, she explains that the ratio of power-to-weight in a competing gymnast is of primary importance, and that keeping weight under control is crucial for female gymnasts. So in addition to constantly modifying her routines to accomodate her increasing height, Nadia had to struggle to keep her weight under control. In spite of this struggle, she continued to win gold medals and championships.

In 1977 Nadia Comaneci again won the overall gold at the European Championships. In 1978 she took a gold medal on the balance beam in the World Championships and retained her overall title at the European Championships. In 1979 she won gold at a competition in England, and for the third time in a row won the European Championships overall gold; this meant that the trophy remained in her permanent possession. She followed this by winning the World Cup gold medals for the vault and floor exercises in Tokyo, Japan. Not bad for a competitor whom the world press kept insisting was all washed up! Her final triumph was at the Olympic Games in Moscow in 1980 where she took gold medals on the balance beam and in the floor exercises.

Also in 1980, Nadia passed the exams for the university to begin her studies to become a coach. She continued competing while beginning her studies, retiring in 1984 just a few weeks before the Los Angeles Olympic games.

Meanwhile, events on the larger stage of world politics were affecting Nadia's life in Bucharest. As the communist regimes in Eastern Europe began to crumble, life in Romania under dictator Nicolae Ceausescu became more and more difficult. The repressive policies of the government allowed less and less personal freedom. Many well-known public figures began to defect to the west, as Bela Karolyi did in 1981 during an exhibition tour of the United States. His relations with the Romanian government had become so tense that he feared for his life.

One result of these defections was that the government kept other sports heroes under constant observation, not allowing them to travel outside of the communist bloc countries. For years Nadia continued in her official government coaching job, until finally she could no longer bear the restrictive policies. In 1989 Nadia Comaneci realized that she would rather die attempting to be free than continue to live in a communist country. Nadia made her way to the Hungarian border and walked six hours in darkness to cross undetected into Hungary. There she was met by the man who helped her escape, Constantin Panait, a former

Romanian who lived in Florida. Panait took her to Vienna, and then to the United States.

Nadia's problems were not over, however. Panait's interest in helping her had been to exploit her fame to make money. They travelled around the country, living in motel rooms while she gave performances and television interviews. Nadia was a virtual prisoner of Panait, who took the money she was paid for her appearances and threatened to have her deported if she complained. She gained weight, and wore heavy make-up to conceal her ill health.

But Nadia's situation was being observed by her friends in the gymnastic community, such as Bart Conner who had last seen her in 1981 during the Romanian team's tour of the United States. Her troubles were also noticed by another Romanian, rugby coach Alexandru Stefu who lived in Montreal. Stefu and other friends invited Panait and Nadia to a meeting, pretending that they could offer a contract for Nadia's performances that would bring in a lot of money. At the meeting they asked Nadia if Panait was mistreating her, and she confessed that he was. Stefu and his family provided a home for Nadia while she lost weight and got back into shape. Later she moved to

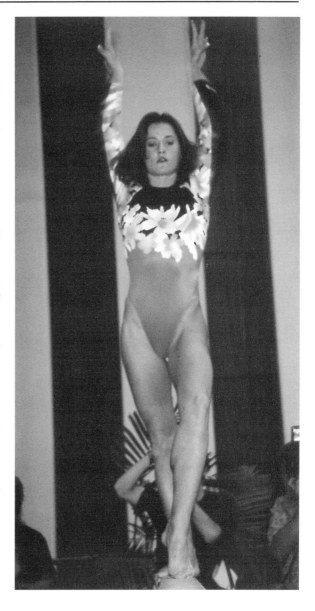

*Nadia served as a spokesperson for the Jockey Underwear Company.*

Oklahoma and took a room in the home of Bart Conner's coach, Paul Ziert, who arranged her gymnastics shows.

Bart Conner is the only American gymnast to win gold medals at every level of national and international competition. He was a Junior National Champion, an Elite National Champion, a World Cup Champion (the only American ever to win a gold medal at a World Cup event), a World Champion, and an Olympic Champion. His accomplishments have been equalled by very few gymnasts in the world, male or female. Of course one of those very few is Nadia Comaneci.

Bart Conner, the 18-year-old gymnast who had shared the American Cup International win with Nadia when she was 14, and who had bent to kiss her as they held their silver cups 15 years before, teamed up with Nadia Comaneci professionally to give gymnastic exhibitions. Before long it was clear that they had teamed up romantically as well. Together they developed the Bart Conner Gymnastics Academy, and together they moved into a beautiful custom-built home in Norman, Oklahoma, in July of 1993.

In November of 1994, five years after Nadia's escape from Romania, and after Ceausescu's regime had been toppled and Romania was a free country, Nadia returned to Romania with Bart for a visit. On their way, while they were in Amsterdam, Bart gave Nadia a diamond ring and proposed. She was so surprised she said, "No," but it took her only a minute to change her mind! They were married on April 27, 1996, in Bucharest, in an ancient Romanian Orthodox Monastery. Young Romanian gymnasts, dressed in leotards, lined the stairs of the church.

When they returned to the United States after their wedding, Nadia and Bart were active in the Olympic Torch ceremonies that began the 1996 Olympic games. Since that time they have continued to be active in promoting and teaching gymnastics, as well as in supporting charity events. In 1998 they agreed to participate in the Legendary Sports Celebrity Roast in Miami to benefit paralysis research at the University of Miami School of Medicine. They have had a regular cable TV show, *Food and Fitness*, in which they share recipes that contribute to good nutrition.

Nadia and Bart write an advice column for Bart's magazine, *International Gymnast*, in which they answer questions sent in by young gymnasts all over the world (their column can also be read on *International Gymnast Online* on the internet). In August of 1999 Nadia took a group of 13 young gymnasts from their Norman, Oklahoma club to Romania to train in Bucharest. Then they visited her hometown of Onesti.

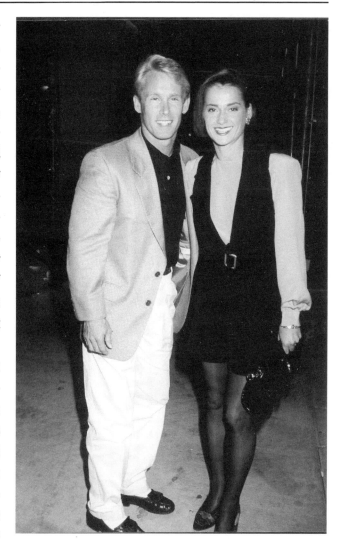

*Bart Conner and Nadia at Caesar's Palace in 1992.*

Nadia Comaneci, and her husband Bart Conner, are working hard to give to the world of gymastics full measure of the challenges and the joys they have received from it.

# Chronology

1961  Born in Onesti, Romania, on November 12

1965  Starts kindergarten in the local public school

1968  Discovered by gymnastics coach Bela Karolyi at the Onesti kindergarten

1969  Finishes 13th in first competition, the National Junior Championships

1970  Wins the National Junior Championships

1971  Wins the Romanian all-around title for her age group; receives gold medals on bars and beam at Friendship Cup in Bulgaria

1973  Wins overall gold at the Friendship Cup competition in East Germany

1975  Wins Champions All competition in England; for the first time, takes overall gold at the European Championships in Skien, Norway

1976  Overall winner at the American Cup in New York; gains fame with seven perfect scores en route to the overall gold at the Montreal Olympic Games

1977  Wins overall gold title at European Championships in Prague, Czechoslovakia

1979  Wins overall gold for the third straight time at the European Championships in Copenhagen, Denmark

1980  Wins Olympic gold medals in beam and floor exercises in Moscow, U.S.S.R.

1981  Admitted to the Sports University in Bucharest

1984  Officially retired from gymnastics competition

1989  Escapes from Romania to the United States

1992  Moves to Norman, Oklahoma, and started giving exhibitions with Bart Conner

1996  Marries Bart Conner in Bucharest, Romania, on April 27

1999   Voted one of the top 25 Outstanding Sports
       People of the Century by the International As-
       sociation of Sports Writers
2000   Participates in Los Angeles County's Parade of
       Nations in February

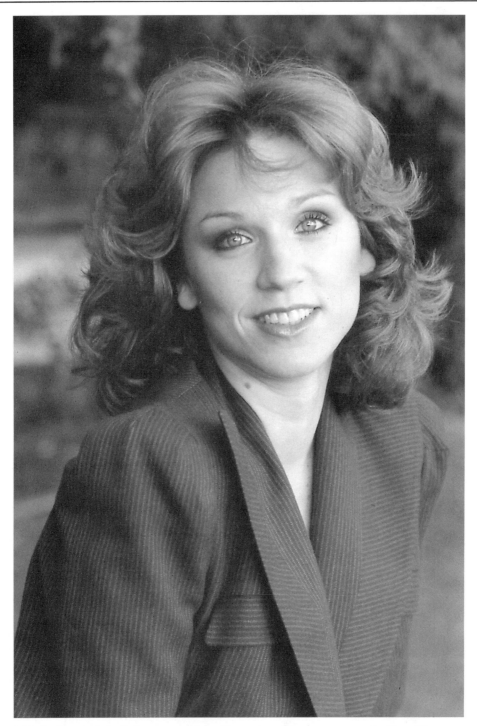

*Marilu Henner's holistic approach to fitness involves every aspect of her life.*

# CHAPTER FIVE
# Marilu Henner

"**H**ealth is not just about weight or appearance, but rather a much bigger picture. I really believe that you can't be a healthy person unless everything is working together. Your body, your mind, your living space," Marilu Henner declares. Her holistic approach to fitness, in which every aspect of a person's life should be involved in achieving good health, is explained in her recent books *Marilu Henner's Total Health Makeover* (1998) and *The 30-Day Total Health Makeover* (1999). "I've met so many people who are looking for something beyond weight loss," Henner says, "to get beyond thinking of 'health' as losing weight in a quick, temporary way."

Marilu was born in Chicago on April 6, 1952, the third of six children. Her father, Joseph, supported his large family by managing car dealerships. Marilu's mother, Loretta, was a dance teacher who ran a performing school at home, giving lessons in her back yard in good weather and in the converted garage in bad weather. The dance studio often turned the Henner household into a gathering place for the whole neighborhood.

Marilu was an active child. She began taking dance lessons from her mother when she was less than three years old, and when she was in fourth grade she and her brothers and sisters appeared in a production of *The King and I*. Marilu says that she was aware at a very young age that she was destined to be a performer, and although her mother encouraged this ambition, her father did not approve.

By the time Marilu was 14, she had become one of the instructors at her mother's dance studio. Some time after that she started participating in local community theater productions. She attended Madonna High, an all-female Catholic school, and in her senior year she had the lead role in a play that dramatized the life of the nun who had founded the school. Her father, who had not encouraged her show business ambitions, was extremely impressed with his daughter's acting skills, and he began to support her efforts to achieve her goal of becoming an actress. Only two weeks later, however, less than a week after Christmas, Joseph Henner died of a heart attack. He was 52.

Despite the loss of her father, Marilu managed to finish her final year in high school. She graduated third in her class, winning an Outstanding American Youth Foundation scholarship in 1970. She used the scholarship to attend the University of Chicago. While there, she ran into Jim Jacobs, an old friend from her community theater days. Jacobs invited her to audition for a production of a musical he was working on called *Grease*, and Marilu took his advice and landed a role. She performed three days a week while carrying her college course load. Jacobs worked on the musical while it was in production, and gradually he developed a more polished, final version. In 1971, he decided that *Grease* was ready for New York, and he asked Marilu to accompany him and stay in the cast. Marilu decided that she wanted to finish college—and the Broadway production of *Grease* took the country by storm and became an enormous hit.

Considering the success of Jacobs's musical, Marilu naturally harbored a few regrets over her decision to stay in Chicago. But in 1972 she got another chance: Jacobs contacted Marilu again, asking her to audition for the touring company of *Grease*. She ended up with the same role she had performed in the Chicago production—and it marked the beginning of her career as a professional performer.

Also in the *Grease* touring company was another young performer who was just breaking into the business—John Travolta. Marilu and John were the youngest members of the company, and they became good friends. At times over the next few years, the friendship turned into an on-again, off-again romance. The two discovered that they had a lot in common: both hailed from large, close-knit Catholic families whose members supported their aspirations. Both knew since childhood that they wanted to perform—and both had the talent, energy, and determination to succeed.

After the *Grease* tour ended, Marilu Henner and John Travolta were both cast in *Over Here*, a World War II–era musical about the singing group known as the Andrews Sisters. Marilu then landed a dancing role in a Broadway production of the musical *Pal Joey*. At the time, Marilu was also getting a lot of parts in television commercials. She knew that to continue a film career she'd probably have to relocate to Los Angeles, California. Finally, in 1977, she did just that. Her first two films were *Between the Lines* and *Bloodbrothers*, a 1978 film costarring Richard Gere. That year she also earned the part of Elaine Nardo in the television sitcom *Taxi*, which centered on a group of taxi drivers who had dreams of leaving their jobs behind and achieving great things.

The character Marilu played—the only woman in the regular cast—was an art dealer by day and a taxi driver by night. Elaine Nardo was one of the most popular characters in the series. The other taxi drivers were played by actors Tony Danza, Judd Hirsch, and Christopher Lloyd, with Danny Devito as their dispatcher. Marilu has since called her years on the cast of *Taxi* "the best experience of my life—the best group of people I've ever worked with." Of course being the only woman gained Marilu lots of attention from her fellow cast members, and she fell in love with them. They, in turn, adored her.

But though Marilu was doing well in her career, her private life was quite different. Just as Marilu was auditioning for *Taxi* in 1978, her mother was stricken with an arthritic condition that damaged her spinal cord. Marilu stayed in Chicago to care for her mother, who died of the ailment two months later. It was the darkest period of Marilu's life. "I watched her suffering in the hospital," Marilu has said, "this strong, vital person who had been teaching dance only a few months before . . . and I thought, 'This shouldn't happen'" In an effort to make sense of what was happening to her mother, Marilu began reading everything she could find about nutrition and health. She also sought out a psychoanalyst to help her understand the mental and emotional components of good health.

On taping breaks from *Taxi*, Marilu continued to work toward a film career. In 1980, while auditioning for a film, she had to kiss an actor named Frederic

Forrest during a scene. She says that she "fell instantly, madly in love" with Forrest at that very moment. Both Marilu and Frederic earned roles in the film, and they got married six months later. The movie, *Hammett*, was a box-office disappointment, however—and before long the marriage was in trouble as well. Forrest was a heavy drinker, and the couple also discovered that they were not very well suited for one another in the long run. Two years later, they divorced.

In 1983–84, Marilu made two movies—*The Man Who Loved Women* and *Cannonball Run II*—with Burt Reynolds, a well-known actor who had become a good friend. "Burt and I had instant chemistry—we just adored each other," Marilu remembered. In 1985 she also appeared in a movie with her old friend John Travolta. Although the movie, which was called *Perfect* and was about the fitness craze, did not do well, the two did have success in another venue: in his book *Staying Fit,* John Travolta featured Marilu in a number of photographs designed to illustrate exercises that partners can do together.

Around the same time, Marilu began seeing director Robert Lieberman. The two had met in 1984, but Marilu was about to leave for Spain to begin filming a movie, and they did not get together again for a year. They both knew right from the start, however, that they seemed to belong together. Still, when Rob asked Marilu to marry him, she turned him down. She told him that she didn't want to repeat the mistake she had once made of marrying too soon. Rob gave her the ring he had bought for her, and told her that should she ever decide that she was ready to marry him, she should just put it on. Soon after, around the time that Marilu appeared in Mike Nichols's Broadway play *Social Secu-*

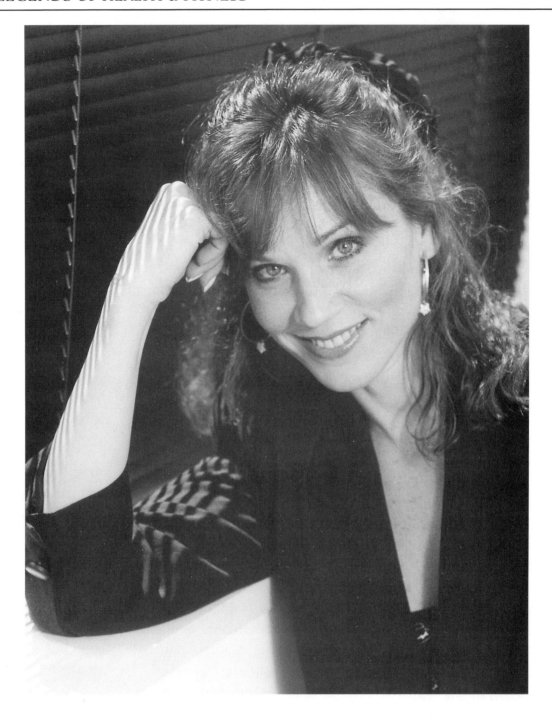

*Marilu starred in* Evening Shade *with Burt Reynolds from 1991 to 1994.*

*rity,* Marilu and Rob began living together. Five years later, Marilu finally put on the engagement ring Rob had given her. The two were married in Italy on June 27, 1990.

That year, Marilu also appeared with Burt Reynolds in the TV series *Evening Shade.* The series was set in a small town in Arkansas, and Reynolds was cast as the coach of the local high school football team; Marilu played his wife. During breaks from filming *Evening Shade,* Marilu continued to act in movies. She appeared in *L.A. Story,* starring comedian Steve Martin, in 1991, and in *Noises Off* in 1992; two years later she had a role in *Chasers.* In 1994–95 she also hosted her own daytime TV talk show, and she published an autobiography, *By All Means Keep on Moving,* in 1994.

Although Marilu and Rob both wanted children, three years passed before they would have the chance. (Marilu jokes that it happened after she repeatedly had to perform a stunt for *Evening Shade* rehearsals, claiming that the activity jostled things around inside.) Nicholas Morgan Lieberman was born on May 12, 1994, to delighted parents. "It took three years because I was waiting for Nicky," Marilu enthused. Nine months later she became pregnant again, and their second son, Joseph Marlon, was born on November 12, 1995.

Although her sons come first in her life, Marilu appears to have boundless energy and enthusiasm, and she continues to perform and to write. She appeared in the television version of *Titanic* in 1996 as the historical character Molly Brown. In 1997 she joined the Broadway revival of the hit musical *Chicago,* after training vigorously to get in shape for the demanding dance role. In 1999, Marilu played herself in the film *Man on the Moon,* based on the life story of her friend, comedian Andy Kaufman, a costar on the *Taxi* series who died in 1984.

In 1998, *Marilu Henner's Total Health Makeover* was published, followed in 1999 by *The 30-Day Total Health Makeover*. Marilu's fitness program is not for the faint of heart or the weak of will. It requires determination and commitment, and she offers no easy promises of quick results with minimum effort. In her program, she challenges many of the habitual ways we behave and consume food. But to the reader Marilu declares, "I would like you to feel really good about facing these challenges. With every step you take, you get one step closer to achieving that ultimate goal of finding a way of life that doesn't deprive you. A way that fills you with the satisfaction of knowing you are treating yourself the way you deserve to be treated—stronger, healthier, and with better clarity both physically and mentally."

*Marilu Henner's Total Health Makeover* outlines 10 steps for a fit and healthy body. Because the program is difficult, she says that some people will be horrified by the effort and may claim that it is impossible to follow. She confesses that she had the same reaction when she first realized that she needed to change her own diet and fitness routine. But she remained so committed and so determined to find a way to prevent the kind of early deaths that took her father and mother that she managed to go on.

Most of the steps in Marilu's program are designed to "detoxify" the body—help it rid itself of an unhealthy buildup of the substances a person has consumed for years. This detoxifying process, she says, sometimes causes uncomfortable symptoms similar to those that people experience when withdrawing from drugs such as nicotine. Step one is primarily an educational process: becoming aware of and eliminating the chemicals, preservatives, and additives that are in most commercially processed foods. "The average consumer eats about 26 pounds of food additives a year," Marilu says. "This should clue you in to the fact that we are putting substances into our bodies that aren't meant to be there. Most of the nearly 3,000 additives used in our food are not considered harmful by the FDA (Food and Drug Administration); however, that doesn't mean that they aren't doing damage to our bodies!"

According to the FDA, an additive is any substance that affects food but is not itself a food. Additives and preservatives keep food from spoiling and give it a longer "shelf life" for the consumer. Marilu admits that it is not possible to completely eliminate additives and preservatives in one's diet, but she believes that it's important to be aware of them and to read labels on the products we buy so that we can try to reduce them. Taking the time and making the effort to seek fresh, organically grown fruits, vegetables, and grains is a cornerstone of this program.

Step two requires eliminating caffeine, a substance that is thought to carry significant health risks and is believed to cause dependency in some users. Caffeine is found not only in coffee and tea but also in chocolate and many soft drinks, as well as in over-the-counter medications such as aspirin and other pain relievers. Most experts would agree with Marilu's recommendation that a person who consumes caffeine should decrease its use gradually to prevent uncomfortable withdrawal symptoms.

Step three of Marilu's plan requires eliminating sugar and sugar substitutes (such as saccharin and aspartame) from the diet. She quotes statistics reporting that the average American eats about 136 pounds of sugar annually, and she lists a number of diseases and ailments that can be worsened by overconsumption of sugars: hyperactivity, diabetes, hypoglycemia, yeast infections, obesity, tooth decay, osteoporosis, and a host of digestive problems. This doesn't mean that one needs to eliminate sugar completely—natural sweeteners, such as raw honey, can easily replace refined sugar in most cases. Products containing maltose, such as rice syrup and barley malt, are also good sugar substitutes.

Step four of Marilu Henner's plan requires that you eliminate meat from your diet. She points out that a great number of health problems are related to eating red meat, including higher risks of various types of cancer, particularly colon cancer. And she says that although her initial goal was to eliminate only red meat from her diet, she now avoids eating chicken, turkey, and other fowl as well. Interestingly enough, she links the elimination of sugar from the diet with the elimination of meat, claiming that refined sugars and red meat are opposite extremes of food, and thus eliminating one will diminish cravings for the other. "Dropping one from the diet makes it easier to stick with not eating either food because your craving for both goes way down," Marilu writes.

Dairy products are not on Marilu's menu either. She has a missionary's fervor about convincing people to stay away from dairy products. "This is my mission— to get the world off dairy products," she says. "I'm always saying that the only thing milk is supposed to do is to turn a 50-pound calf into a 300-pound cow in six months. If cows don't drink milk why would we?" To replace dairy products, including yogurt, cheese, sour

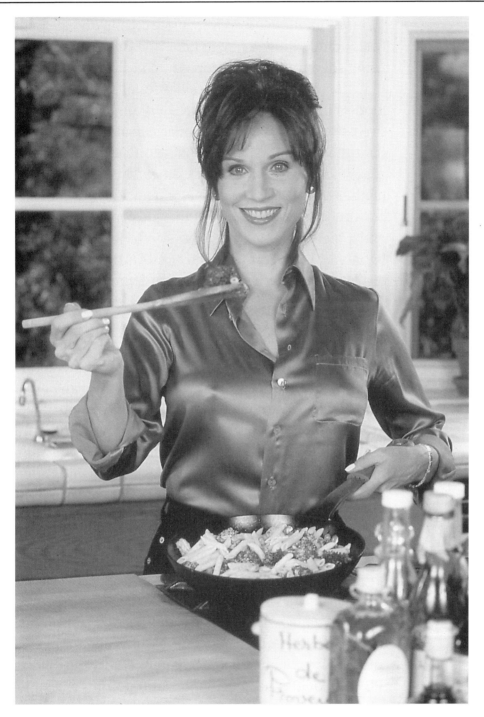

*Fresh, organically grown fruits and vegetables are the cornerstone of Marilu's combining plan.*

cream, creamy salad dressings, ice cream, and all foods that include them as ingredients, Marilu recommends using soy products. In step six, Marilu recommends food combining. It may seem, after all of the types of foods she has eliminated, that not many would be left to combine. But Marilu categorizes meals as fruit, starch (carbohydrates), or protein meals. One should never eat proteins and starches, together, she says, because neither would be properly digested. Eat fruits alone, but do not combine acidic fruits—citrus, strawberries, and pineapples, for example—with sweet fruits like bananas, dates, prunes, and figs. And never eat melons with other types of food, even other fruit.

The concept of food combining requires that one wait several hours after consuming one type of meal before having another type. For example, wait two hours after a fruit meal, three hours after a starch meal, and four hours after a protein meal before having any other kind of meal. Marilu's own choice is to have a fruit meal in the morning, an energy-packed protein meal for lunch, and a starch meal in the evening. In food combining, one can also eat vegetables or fats with a protein or a starch meal.

Marilu's seventh step in her 10-step diet plan is to be aware of the various types of fats: saturated, monounsaturated, and polyunsaturated. Of these, you should avoid those in the first category because they are highest in cholesterol, which can clog blood vessels and cause heart attacks and strokes. All animal fats—those found in meat, poultry, and dairy products—are saturated fats. Cocoa butter and coconut oil are also saturated fats. The monounsaturated fats are somewhat healthier and include olive oil, peanut oil, and canola oil. They are also found in peanut butter and

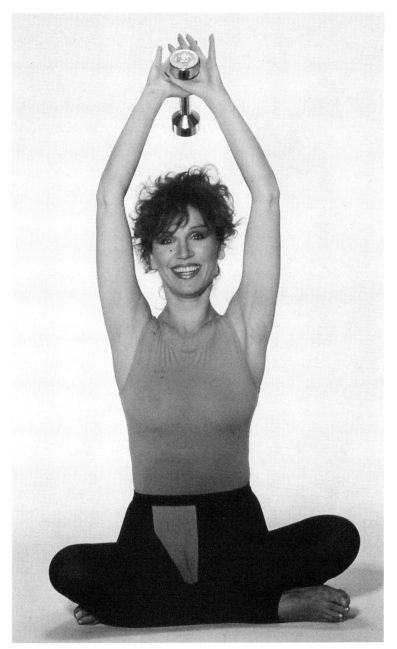

*Marilu considers exercise an absolutely essential part of any successful fitness program.*

avocados. The third group, polyunsaturated fats, are the healthiest, and they are found in some types of fish, as well as soy, corn, sunflower, and safflower oils.

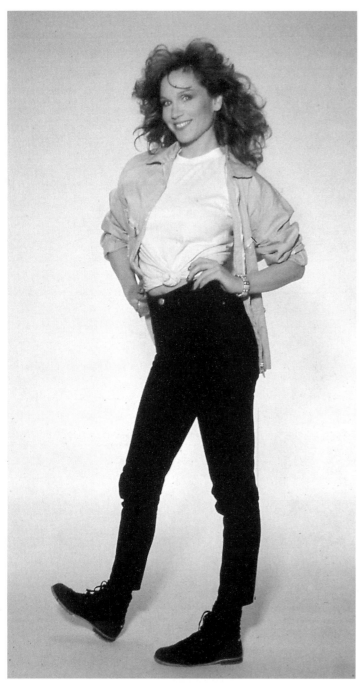

*Marilu combines a positive attitude with everything she does.*

Nutritional experts agree that some fat in the diet is necessary, and they recommend consuming between 20 and 30 percent of your total calorie intake in fats. Marilu cautions against being taken in by the current emphasis on fat-free foods. Many of these foods contain extra sugar and other flavorings to compensate for the absence of fat, and they may also contain more calories. Therefore, they end up being more fattening than the same food would be if it included fat. The best course of action, Marilu says, is not to eliminate fat, but to replace saturated fats with polyunsaturated fats.

Marilu's step eight is exercise, an absolutely essential part of any successful fitness program. "I originally wanted to design an exercise program that would give you some specific routines to develop and follow," she explains, "but I soon realized that exercise is different from all the other components in this program because everyone must approach it in an individual way." She does have one specific requirement: have fun. "Isn't it amazing that it's hard to get a child to stop playing and even harder to get an adult to start?" she says. "There are hundreds of ways to exercise. Find the ones that you will truly look forward to doing every day." Not only should exercise be enjoyable, but it should be varied so that you avoid becoming bored and discouraged. The only other requirement is that you break a sweat for at least 20 to 30 minutes every day. This, she says, will indicate that the body is burning fat.

Step nine in the program is to stay well-rested. Marilu emphasizes, "Getting enough sleep allows your body to be a natural healer for almost every ailment." The body has a built-in regulator, an inner clock, that measures how much sleep it needs, and if it is deprived of that amount it will gradually become run down. How much sleep do we need? It varies with each individual. Some people are refreshed after only six hours of sleep each night; some find that they need 10 to function at their best. It isn't a moral issue, Marilu stresses; it's a question of what your own body needs.

Marilu Henner calls her final step in the program "Gusto." The term has more to do with attitude than with any specific exercises or behaviors. Most people unknowingly put limitations on themselves because of their attitudes toward fitness and exercise. "What happens too often is that we become so discouraged with the distance between where we're at and where we want to be that we give up the fight," she says. "The idea behind Gusto is to break those self-imposed barriers."

Marilu Henner's philosophy of total health goes beyond diet and exercise to challenge "self-imposed barriers" in all aspects of life. She believes that one's surroundings should reflect order and harmony. *The 30-Day Total Health Makeover* not only contains recipes for the foods in her program, but it also includes tips for organizing one's household and clothing, as well as beauty and budget suggestions.

One of Marilu Henner's typical examples to explain her approach to life centers around a term she devised from her experience of growing up in a large family. She said it was "like living in a hamper." The word "hamper," used as an adjective, would describe anything that was not in perfect condition, such as a blouse with a button missing, a sweater with a small hole in it, a stained necktie, or a shoe with a run-down heel. Marilu believes that it's important not to accept such "hamper" items as good enough. Sew on the button, mend the hole, remove the stain, have the shoe repaired. In other words, insist on keeping higher standards not only when it comes to your health, but in every other aspect of your life.

# Chronology

1952  Born on April 6 in Chicago, Illinois
1966  Attends Madonna High School; teaches at her mother's dance studio
1969  Father dies of a heart attack on New Year's Eve
1970  Wins Outstanding American Youth Foundation scholarship; attends University of Chicago; performs in *Grease*
1972  Begins touring in *Grease* with John Travolta
1974  Appears in Broadway musical *Over There*
1977  Moves to Los Angeles
1978  Appears in *Between the Lines* and *Bloodbrothers;* cast as Elaine Nardo in TV sitcom *Taxi;* mother dies
1983  Appears in *The Man Who Loved Women* with Burt Reynolds and *Hammett* with Frederic Forrest; marries Forrest
1984  Appears in *Cannonball Run II* with Burt Reynolds
1985  Appears in *Perfect* with John Travolta; divorces Frederic Forrest
1990  Marries Robert Lieberman; lands role in *Evening Shade*
1991  Appears in *L.A. Story* with Steve Martin
1992  Appears in film version of *Noises Off*
1994  Appears in *Chasers;* publishes autobiography *By All Means Keep on Moving*
1994  Son Nicholas Morgan born on May 12
1995  Son Joseph Marlon born on November 12
1996  Appears in TV movie *Titanic*
1997  Joins cast of Broadway hit musical *Chicago*
1998  Publishes *Marilu Henner's Total Health Makeover*
1999  Publishes *The 30-Day Total Health Makeover;* plays herself in *Man on the Moon*

# Further Reading

Calkins, Laurel Brubaker. "10 Again." *People Weekly* 46, no. 3 (15 July 1996): 65–71

Comaneci, Nadia. *Nadia: The Autobiography of Nadia Comaneci.* New York: Proteus Books, 1981.

Diamond, Jamie. "Chrissy, Incorporated." *Ladies Home Journal* 115, no. 5 (May 1998): 92–94.

Gates, Anita. "Unstoppable Oprah." *McCall's* 127, no. 5 (February 2000): 16.

Gerosa, Melina. "Oprah: Fit for Life." *Ladies Home Journal* 113, no. 2 (February 1996): 108–11

Hallman, Charlie. "Perfect in the Past, Comaneci Sees a Brighter Future." *St. Paul Pioneer Press* (11 April 1996): K-4.

Henner, Marilu, and Jim Jerome. *By All Means Keep on Moving.* New York: Pocket Books, 1994.

Henner, Marilu, and Laura Morton. *The 30 Day Total Health Makeover: Everything You Need to Do to Change Your Body, Your Health, and Your Life in 30 Amazing Days.* New York: HarperCollins, 1999.

———. *Marilu Henner's Total Health Makeover: 10 Steps to Your B.E.S.T. Body: Balance, Energy, Stamina, Toxin-Free.* New York: HarperCollins, 1998.

Modderno, Craig. "Suzanne Somers Gets To the Bottom of Things." *TV Guide* 44, no. 4 (27 January 1996): 8.

Nicholson, Lois P. *Oprah Winfrey.* New York: Chelsea House, 1994.

Smith, Olivia Jane. "Marilu Henner." *Current Biography* 60, no. 2 (February 1999): 23–25.

Somers, Suzanne. *After the Fall: How I Picked Myself Up, Dusted Myself Off, and Started All Over Again.* New York: Crown Publishing, 1998.

———. *Eat Great, Lose Weight.* New York: Crown Publishing, 1997.

———. *Get Skinny on Fabulous Food.* New York: Crown Publishing, 1999.

———. *365 Ways to Change Your Life.* New York: Crown Publishing, 1999.

Taraborrelli, J. Randy. "How Oprah Does It All: The Top-Rated Talk Show, the Grueling Workouts, the Movie Deals, the Social Life, It's Not Just Good Luck. Here's How She Pulls It Off." *Redbook* 187, no. 4 (August 1996): 76–80.

Winfrey, Oprah, and Bob Greene. *Make the Connection: 10 Steps to a Better Body—and a Better Life.* New York: Hyperion, 1996.

# Index